CHIEF COMPLAINT

STORIES AND LESSONS FROM THE FRONTLINES OF MEDICAL CODING

GOLI SAI PHANI

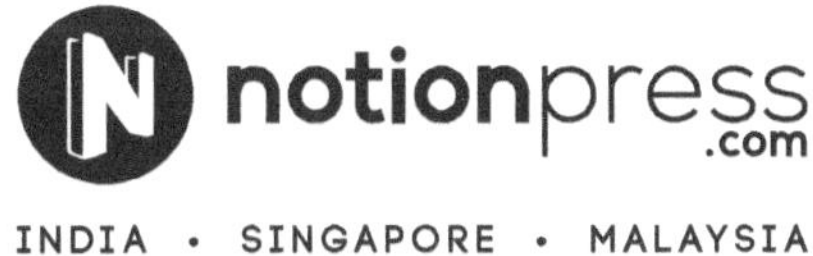

INDIA • SINGAPORE • MALAYSIA

ISBN
Paperback 979-8-89632-449-2
Hardcase 979-8-89632-824-7

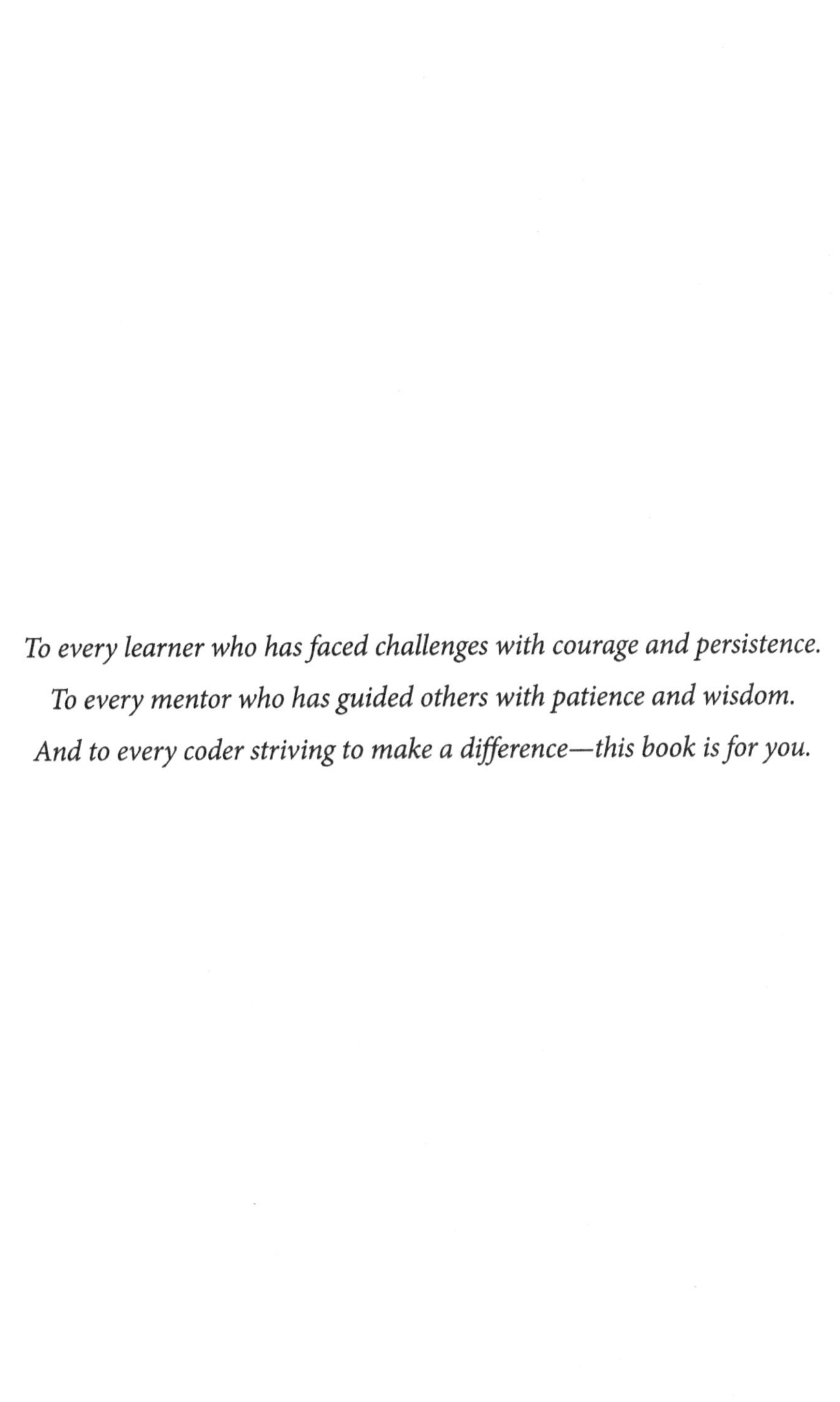

To every learner who has faced challenges with courage and persistence.

To every mentor who has guided others with patience and wisdom.

And to every coder striving to make a difference—this book is for you.

Foreword

Medical coding is often seen as a meticulous and technical task, yet few recognize its profound impact on the healthcare industry. Behind every accurate code lies the story of a patient, a provider's effort, and the coder's skill in translating these narratives into actionable data. "Chief Complaint" is more than just a book—it is a guide, a mentor, and a friend to coders navigating this dynamic field.

When I first encountered Goli Sai Phani's work in the medical coding community, what struck me was not only his expertise but also his passion for teaching. His ability to simplify complex concepts and connect with learners has made him a respected figure in this field. This book is an extension of that dedication, offering insights that are as practical as they are inspiring.

"Chief Complaint" takes a refreshing approach, using relatable stories and actionable lessons to address the challenges coders face daily. Whether you're just stepping into the world of medical coding or looking to refine your skills, this book offers clarity, motivation, and a road map for success.

I encourage you to treat this book not just as a resource but as a companion in your journey. Goli Sai Phani's stories and lessons will guide you through the nuances of coding with precision, confidence, and integrity.

With each chapter, you'll find yourself not just learning but growing—both as a coder and as a professional. Welcome to the next chapter of your medical coding journey.

Warm regards,

Adilakshmi Sankara MBA, CPC, CPC-I, CIC, CRC, CPMA, CCS

Contents

Prologue

To Every Medical Coder, Fresh and Seasoned

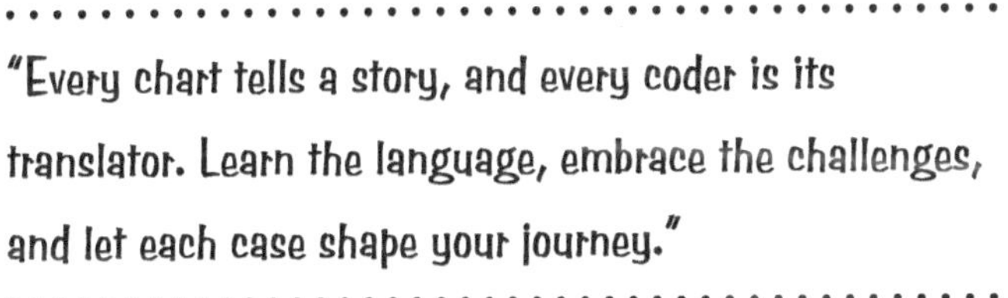

When I first stepped into the world of medical coding, I quickly learned that there was much more to it than the codes themselves. Coding wasn't just about precision; it was about understanding each detail and making decisions that impacted patient care, compliance, and financial integrity. I made my fair share of mistakes, but each one taught me a lesson I never forgot.

This book, *Chief Complaint*, was born from those early lessons and countless stories I've encountered since—both my own and from others in our field. It's written as a guide, a mentor, and a friend to coders navigating similar challenges. You'll find stories of struggle, learning, and triumph, each shared with the hope that you'll find a bit of your own journey here, too.

You may be a fresh graduate eager to get started or a seasoned coder looking to revisit the basics with fresh insight. Wherever you are, my hope is that these stories will resonate, motivate, and remind you that every challenge is an opportunity to grow.

So, let's embark on this journey together. Each chapter, like a "chief complaint," addresses real issues we face in coding and offers insights that can make your path a little smoother. I'm grateful to have you here, and I'm excited for the lessons we'll uncover together.

Welcome to *Chief Complaint*. Let's get started.

– Goli Sai Phani

Acknowledgment

Writing this book has been a journey shaped by the contributions of many people, and I am deeply grateful for their support and encouragement.

To my family, thank you for your unwavering belief in me and for providing the strength to see this project through.

To my mentors and colleagues, your insights, feedback, and guidance have been invaluable in shaping my understanding and my voice.

To my students, you are the inspiration behind this book. Your curiosity, determination, and successes remind me daily of the importance of growth and learning.

Finally, to the medical coding community—thank you for the work you do every day and for being a constant source of inspiration. This book exists because of you and for you.

Introduction

Why "Chief Complaint"?

> "The chief complaint isn't just a clinical detail—it's the spark that sets the entire story in motion. In coding, as in life, understanding the core problem leads to clarity."

Welcome! If you're picking up this book, chances are you've got a healthy curiosity—or perhaps a serious "chief complaint" of your own—about medical coding. Whether you're just starting out, already working in the field, or looking to polish your skills, you're in the right place.

I chose "Chief Complaint" as the title because it's such a fitting metaphor for what we face as medical coders every day. In medical terms, the "chief complaint" is the reason a patient comes to see the doctor, the issue that needs attention right away. But what if we think of each coding challenge as a "chief complaint" in its own right? It's the part of our job that demands problem-solving, precision, and a solid understanding of coding rules and medical nuances. This book is built around that idea: we'll tackle coding challenges like a doctor would a patient's main concern—step by step, examining all the parts, until we arrive at a solution.

What Is a "Chief Complaint," Anyway?

In medical coding, the "chief complaint" is the primary reason the patient is seeking care, whether it's a sore throat, a nagging cough, or persistent chest pain. It's usually the first piece of information you'll come across in a patient's chart, setting the stage for everything that follows. For us as coders, the chief complaint isn't just a casual observation; it drives the diagnosis and impacts the codes that end up on the claim, affecting treatment and billing. In other words, it's critical that we get it right.

But sometimes, the chief complaint isn't straightforward. Maybe the patient describes vague symptoms, or there's more than one reason they came in that day. Similarly, in coding, we often face murky or multi-faceted "complaints" that need our attention, whether it's a complex set of symptoms, incomplete documentation, or deciding between similar codes. Just like a clinician can't jump to a diagnosis without a clear understanding of the complaint, we can't select a code without fully understanding the problem in front of us.

My "Chief Complaint" Moment: Learning from Mistakes

Let me share a story with you. Early in my career, I was working on a seemingly simple case involving abdominal pain. It should've been a straightforward process: read the documentation, code the diagnosis, double-check, and move on. But I rushed, and, without digging deeper, I coded it as generic abdominal pain (R10.9). Later, when the case was reviewed, my supervisor flagged it. "Did you notice the reference to 'RLQ tenderness'?" she asked.

Now, if you're new, "RLQ" stands for "right lower quadrant" of the abdomen, an area often associated with appendicitis. Turns out, I had missed a critical clue. By overlooking that detail, I had missed a more specific diagnosis code that would have better reflected the patient's condition. It was an eye-opener for me—not only about the importance of reading documentation thoroughly but also about how each case has its own "chief complaint," a main challenge or detail that requires our attention.

That experience taught me two big lessons: first, to respect the details (always!), and second, to understand that every coding challenge has its own "chief complaint"—the specific problem or clue that needs our attention. And if you learn to spot and address those "complaints" correctly, you'll get closer to coding mastery.

Treat Each Chapter as a "Consult" for Coding Challenges

Think of this book as a series of consults. Each chapter will focus on a particular challenge or tricky area in medical coding—the kinds of things you might have questions about or wish someone had explained to you sooner. Just like a clinician would consult a specialist for a second opinion, consider these chapters as a way to dive deeper and get practical insights on common (and not-so-common) coding problems. Together, we'll break down each challenge and work through it step by step.

For example, one chapter might focus on deciphering complex cases in emergency medicine, where patients often present with multiple symptoms and vague complaints. Another chapter will look at handling chronic conditions that can impact coding decisions in ways that aren't always obvious at first glance.

And just like in a real consult, I want to give you the kind of practical, hands-on advice that will make coding feel less daunting and more intuitive. I won't be just listing coding rules or guidelines here; I'll walk you through examples, real-life tips, and memorable stories so that you can see how these strategies come alive in day-to-day coding.

Why This Approach Matters for Medical Coders

Medical coding can sometimes feel like a never-ending to-do list: you review the documentation, identify key details, choose codes, review for accuracy, submit the claim, and move on to the next case. It's easy to get lost in the process, and just as easy to overlook that crucial "chief complaint" that each case holds. But once you train yourself to zero in on the main issue in every coding scenario, you'll feel more confident, make fewer errors, and find yourself working faster and smarter.

In fact, this approach is exactly how some of the best coders work: they focus on the most important elements first, understanding that each case presents its own unique coding puzzle. They listen closely to the documentation, just like a clinician listens to a patient. And they prioritize accuracy, knowing that even a single code can affect everything from patient care to reimbursement.

Here's What You'll Learn

Throughout this book, you'll pick up practical skills and insights on coding different types of "complaints"—from specific diagnosis codes to intricate procedures. We'll cover everything from handling uncertain diagnoses and coding for chronic conditions to working with encounter notes and understanding the nuances of surgical codes.

Each chapter will give you tools to break down coding challenges and help you find your way through complex cases.

You'll also learn how to navigate those gray areas where the coding guidelines aren't black and white, and we'll go over strategies for reading between the lines in clinical notes. Coding is an art as much as a science, and just like any art form, it improves with practice, insight, and a bit of confidence.

Why You Can Trust Yourself to Do This

If you're new to coding or if you've ever second-guessed your work, know that you're not alone. Every coder, no matter how experienced, has had moments of doubt or made mistakes. It's all part of the learning process. The key is to build up your knowledge and practice noticing those "chief complaints" in your work.

So, here's my challenge to you as you read: treat each chapter as a hands-on experience. Make notes, try out the strategies on real cases if you can, and see how you can apply each lesson. Coding can feel overwhelming, but every bit of insight you gain makes you a stronger coder. You're learning a skill that combines knowledge, logic, and care for detail—so every improvement counts

Final Thoughts: Let's Get Started

This book is here to support you on your journey, no matter where you're starting. Just remember, each coding challenge is like a chief complaint. It's a chance to improve, get creative, and learn a little more every day. By the end, my hope is that you'll feel empowered to take on any coding problem with confidence and a clear plan of action.

Now, let's dive in and start solving these coding complaints together. You're already on the right path, and I'm here to guide you every step of the way!

Chapter 1

First Encounters

> "The first step into any field is like entering a maze. It's confusing, overwhelming, and sometimes disheartening—but every wrong turn teaches you how to find your way."

Welcome to the world of medical coding! Whether you're brand new to coding or have a little experience under your belt, it's safe to say that those first few days can be a bit overwhelming. The sheer number of codes, the medical terminology, and the documentation you're expected to read and interpret can all feel like an avalanche of information.

But you're not alone, and the feelings you're having are entirely normal. Nearly every coder has had that "first day" experience—a blend of excitement, nerves, and a sense of "Am I really ready for this?"

Let's talk about why these first encounters with medical coding are so foundational to everything that follows.

First Day on the Job: A Personal Story

My own first day in medical coding is a story I still share with newcomers because it was a real eye-opener. I remember walking into the coding department, feeling pretty confident. I'd done my training, knew the basics, and felt ready to dive in. Then, my manager handed me a thick stack of charts and told me to code them as practice before submitting anything. I started flipping through, and it was like stepping into a whole new language.

The charts were full of medical jargon, diagnoses that seemed to have endless variations, and a bunch of shorthand and acronyms I had never seen before. For instance, I saw "CHF" and "COPD" and initially had no idea how they differed or what nuances were hiding within them. The codes seemed like an endless maze, and even simple diagnoses like "diabetes" came with layers of detail.

Within the first hour, I felt completely lost. I'd made mistakes, felt unsure about each step, and had questions I wasn't sure I wanted to ask. But I quickly learned that asking questions was the key to learning. I went to my manager and asked for guidance, and that was when things started to click. We reviewed a chart together, broke it down piece by piece, and I saw how each term, abbreviation, and code played a specific role.

Why Accuracy Matters Right from the Start

Medical coding might seem like just "entering the right codes" at first glance, but the role is far more significant. Every code you choose represents a real person's health journey and impacts both their care and the healthcare provider's reimbursement. Small inaccuracies, like selecting the wrong code for a patient's condition, can lead to complications down the road. For instance, if you accidentally choose a generic diagnosis code instead of a more specific one, it can affect the level of care the patient receives, the physician's revenue, or even compliance with insurance guidelines.

Accuracy isn't about perfection—it's about taking the time to check your work, verify details, and ensure the codes you select truly represent the patient's health status. While mistakes are part of the learning process, the goal is to approach every chart with care and to grow more confident with each case.

Detail is Your Best Friend

In coding, details make all the difference. For instance, let's take a common condition like "diabetes." Did you know that there are over a dozen codes just for diabetes alone? And each code reflects different complications, types, and control levels. It's easy to see why attention to detail is critical! The more you tune into the specifics—like which type of diabetes the patient has and whether it's well-controlled or not—the more precise your coding will be.

Think of the chart like a puzzle: each symptom, each diagnosis, and each treatment are clues that lead you to the right codes. And just like any puzzle, you won't solve it by glancing over the details. It's often in the small things—the patient's specific complaints, the treatments noted, or the diagnostic findings—where you'll find the keys to coding accurately.

A quick way to build your "detail muscle": Practice reading charts slowly and focus on understanding each word. Take the time to look up any unfamiliar terms or diagnoses. Every term you learn and understand helps you tackle future cases more effectively.

Overcoming the Initial Fears

It's perfectly natural to feel intimidated or even afraid of making mistakes. Coding is a field where precision is rewarded, and it can feel overwhelming to get everything right from the start. But the beauty of medical coding is that it's a skill, and like any skill, it gets better with practice. Every coder you see confidently handling charts and codes once stood exactly where you are now.

Here are a few tips to ease those initial fears:

1. **Ask for Guidance**: The best coders are often those who aren't afraid to ask questions. Find a mentor or a more experienced coder who can help answer questions or review tricky cases with you.
2. **Take It One Step at a Time**: Coding isn't a race. Especially in the beginning, focus on taking each chart as it comes. Break it down, review the details, and don't rush. Speed will come with time.
3. **Learn from Feedback**: Early on, you'll probably receive feedback on your coding. Rather than seeing corrections as mistakes, view them as learning opportunities. Every time you make a correction, you're sharpening your skills and gaining knowledge.
4. **Give Yourself Time**: Coding is like learning a new language; it requires patience and persistence. Trust that you'll get better every day, and allow yourself to make (and learn from) mistakes.

Getting Comfortable with Coding Guidelines

One of the first things you'll encounter in coding is a set of guidelines. It may feel like there's an overwhelming amount of rules, but these guidelines are actually a coder's best friend. They exist to guide you in making the best choices for each patient case and help ensure that coding is consistent and accurate across the board.

Start by focusing on the core guidelines, like those around diagnoses and principal procedures. These will become the foundation for much of your coding work, especially in cases involving multiple complaints or complex diagnoses. As you get more comfortable, branch out and explore more specialized guidelines, like those specific to certain procedures or chronic conditions.

A **quick way to approach guidelines**: Try creating a cheat sheet for yourself with the top 5–10 most important points. This can act as a quick reference until you're more comfortable with the details. Over time, you'll remember these intuitively, but at the beginning, having a quick reference can be a lifesaver.

Practice with Purpose

When you're new, it's essential to get hands-on practice with actual cases or mock charts. Reading about coding is great, but the real learning happens when you work with real-life examples. If your workplace offers practice charts, take advantage of them. If not, try finding sample charts or case studies that you can practice coding on your own.

Each time you complete a chart, take a moment to review it and double-check your work. Look for opportunities to apply what you've learned about accuracy, detail, and guidelines. The more you practice with purpose, the faster you'll build your confidence.

Remember, every coding session is a chance to learn: Each chart you code, whether it's simple or complex, is building your skills. Take each coding task seriously, and use it as an opportunity to apply what you're learning in real time.

Wrapping Up: Your First Steps Matter

Starting your career in medical coding is a big step, and every experience you have along the way adds to your growth. Right now, everything may feel new and challenging, but know that each case you code is getting you closer to becoming a skilled, confident coder.

Remember, every seasoned coder started as a beginner, fumbling through their first charts and learning from mistakes. You're on the same path, and each day brings you closer to expertise. You've chosen a profession that requires detail, care, and a commitment to accuracy—qualities that make you a vital part of the healthcare team.

As you keep going, stay curious, be patient with yourself, and remember to celebrate the small victories. You're doing great, and each case, question, and correction is another step forward.

Chapter 2

Lost in Translation – Understanding the Language of Coding

"Every new language feels foreign at first. But with patience and practice, what once seemed like chaos becomes second nature."

If you're new to medical coding, you've probably noticed that it feels like learning a new language. And that's because, in a way, it is! Medical coding is filled with terminology and shorthand that can seem overwhelming at first, and just like any language, it comes with its own vocabulary, grammar, and quirks.

In this chapter, we'll tackle some of the common "lost in translation" moments that come with medical coding, and I'll share tips to make this language feel more like second nature.

Lost in Translation: My First Encounter with Medical Jargon

Let's start with a little story from my early days. I remember sitting down with my first real batch of charts, ready to code away, only to get stuck on terms like "TIA," "hypoxemia," and "bronchospasm." Each one sounded like a puzzle. I'd skim through the documentation trying to find clues, but it felt like a maze of unfamiliar words, abbreviations, and phrases.

At one point, I came across the term "TIA," which I coded as "transient ischemic attack." Later, I learned that TIA often presents with symptoms that could look like other conditions, so context matters. It turns out that understanding the broader context of terms and conditions isn't just helpful—it's crucial. Each word can affect the coding outcome, and sometimes, tiny details make a big difference in how you approach a case.

Building Your Medical Vocabulary: The Core Concepts

Medical coding has a set of core concepts that appear across many charts and cases. If you understand these basics, you'll find that other terms start to make sense more quickly. Let's dive into some of the most common categories of terms you'll see in coding.

1. Anatomical Terms

Knowing the human body's basic anatomy will help you immediately spot what part of the body is involved. For example, if you see terms like "cranial," "thoracic," or "renal," you're dealing with the head, chest, and kidneys, respectively. Here's a quick breakdown of some commonly used anatomical terms:

- **Cranial** – Relating to the skull
- **Thoracic** – Refers to the chest area
- **Abdominal** – The area of the stomach
- **Cervical** – Relating to the neck
- **Femoral** – Refers to the thigh area

Tip for learning anatomical terms: Get a simple diagram of the body and label these common areas with the terms you come across most often. It's like your own mini map, helping you learn to navigate the body's terrain.

2. Diagnostic Terms

Diagnosis terms reflect a patient's condition and can be specific or general. These are the words that describe illnesses, injuries, and conditions. Terms like "hypertension," "diabetes," "hypoxemia," and "cholecystitis" will come up again and again. Each diagnosis has nuances, so here's a quick breakdown of some common ones:

- **Hypertension** – High blood pressure; often specified as "essential" or "secondary."
- **Hypoxemia** – Low oxygen levels in the blood.

- **Cholecystitis** – Inflammation of the gallbladder.
- **Myocardial infarction** – A heart attack; look for terms like "acute" and "non-ST elevation."

A practical trick: When you encounter a new diagnostic term, jot it down along with a quick definition. Try to use it in context on your next practice chart. Repetition will help these terms stick.

3. Symptomatic Terms

Symptoms are often the starting point for a diagnosis and can guide you to the right codes. Here are a few common ones:

- **Dyspnea** – Shortness of breath.
- **Syncope** – Fainting or passing out.
- **Hematuria** – Blood in the urine.
- **Edema** – Swelling, often due to fluid accumulation.

Quick tip: If you're faced with symptomatic terms, pair them with possible diagnostic terms. For example, dyspnea might lead you to conditions like asthma, pneumonia, or congestive heart failure.

Decoding Medical Abbreviations

Abbreviations are a big part of the "language of coding." They're a convenient shorthand, but if you don't know them, they can slow you down. Here are a few to get you started:

- **COPD** – Chronic obstructive pulmonary disease.
- **CHF** – Congestive heart failure.
- **MI** – Myocardial infarction (heart attack).
- **UTI** – Urinary tract infection.
- **CVA** – Cerebrovascular accident (stroke).
- **TIA** – Transient ischemic attack (mini-stroke).

Making Sense of Medical Prefixes and Suffixes

Breaking down complex medical terms can make them feel less intimidating. Most terms have a prefix (beginning), root (middle), and suffix (end) that describe what's going on. Here's a quick guide:

- **Prefixes**: These usually indicate location, time, or amount. For example:
  - ☐ **Hypo**- means "low" or "under," as in **hypoglycemia** (low blood sugar).
  - ☐ **Hyper**- means "high" or "above," as in **hypertension** (high blood pressure).
  - ☐ **Brady**- means "slow," as in **bradycardia** (slow heart rate).
- **Roots**: The core part of the word that usually refers to a body part. For example:
  - ☐ **Cardi**- refers to the heart (e.g., **cardiology**).
  - ☐ **Neuro**- refers to nerves (e.g., **neurology**).
  - ☐ **Osteo**- refers to bones (e.g., **osteoporosis**).
- **Suffixes**: These often indicate a condition or procedure. For example:
  - ☐ **itis** means "inflammation," as in **arthritis** (inflammation of the joints).
  - ☐ **ectomy** means "removal of," as in **appendectomy** (removal of the appendix).
  - ☐ **scopy** means "to view or examine," as in **colonoscopy** (examination of the colon).

Takeaway: If a term seems confusing, try breaking it down into parts. Recognizing prefixes, roots, and suffixes will give you clues about its meaning.

Practice Strategies for Learning Medical Terms

Mastering the language of coding takes time, but here are a few tips to help you along the way.

1. **Create Flashcards**: Old-school flashcards can work wonders! Write the term on one side and the definition on the other, and flip through them daily. Digital apps can work, too, if you prefer something you can carry on your phone.
2. **Use Mnemonics**: Mnemonics are memory aids, and they're great for memorizing medical terms. For example, to remember "COPD," you might think, "Can't Overcome Pulmonary Disease." Get creative with these!
3. **Use Context to Build Your Knowledge**: Try to read short medical case summaries or sample charts. Focus on identifying the main terms and translating them. With regular practice, you'll start to recognize patterns and terms more easily.
4. **Review Common Conditions**: Some conditions pop up repeatedly in coding, so it's a good idea to get familiar with them early on. Spend some time reading up on common diagnoses like hypertension, diabetes, and heart disease.

Avoiding Common Language Mistakes

When you're new, it's easy to misinterpret terms or overlook critical details. Here are a few common language pitfalls to watch for:

- **Mistaking Similar-Sounding Terms**: Terms like "hypoglycemia" (low blood sugar) and "hyperglycemia" (high blood sugar) look almost identical but mean the opposite. Always double-check if you're unsure.
- **Overlooking Modifiers**: Certain words, like "acute" and "chronic," can significantly alter the diagnosis. "Chronic" conditions are long-term, while "acute" refers to something sudden or severe. Coding these accurately impacts both the treatment path and reimbursement.
- **Ignoring Context**: Medical terms can have different meanings depending on context. For instance, "chronic pain" is different from "acute pain," and each one has specific coding requirements.

A practical tip: If you're unsure about a term, look it up and see if there's an example case that uses it. Understanding how a term is used in context can help you avoid common misunderstandings.

Wrapping Up: You're Learning a New Skill—Be Patient!

Medical coding language isn't something you master overnight. Just like learning a spoken language, it requires time, practice, and exposure. Each term you learn, each abbreviation you decode, and each case you work through brings you one step closer to fluency.

As you keep learning, remember that no one expects you to know every term right away. If you encounter new language, take a deep breath, break it down, and trust that every small effort adds to your understanding. You're building a skill that will make you an invaluable part of any healthcare team.

Stay curious, keep practicing, and remember—every coder has felt "lost in translation" at some point. You're doing great, and every term you learn is a win.

Chapter 3

Guideline Blindness – Ignoring Conventions and Guidelines

"Guidelines aren't rules to limit you—they're the framework that turns uncertainty into precision. Ignore them, and you're coding blind."

Medical coding is full of rules, conventions, and guidelines that aren't just there to make life difficult—they're there to ensure accuracy, consistency, and compliance. As tempting as it can be to skim or even skip these guidelines when you're deep in a chart, doing so can lead to errors that affect everything from reimbursement to patient care.

In this chapter, we'll dig into what I like to call "guideline blindness"—the tendency to overlook or bypass coding guidelines. I'll share a story from my own experience to highlight just how important these rules are, and then we'll break down some of the core guidelines to show why they matter.

The Hard Way: Learning Why Guidelines Matter

Early on, I had an experience that taught me the importance of following coding guidelines, even when they seem trivial. I was coding a case involving a patient with diabetes and an eye complication. In my rush to wrap up, I picked what I thought was the correct code for diabetic retinopathy, without double-checking the guidelines. It wasn't until later that I learned I'd overlooked a major guideline that required a secondary code to capture the specific type of complication.

When my coding manager reviewed the chart, she flagged my error, and the case had to be corrected. In addition to the extra work involved, it was a humbling experience that made me realize just how important it is to take guidelines seriously. From that day forward, I made it a rule to consult the guidelines first—no exceptions.

Why Guidelines Are Your Best Friend in Coding

Guidelines are like the GPS for coding. They guide you through the complexities of each case and help you make decisions based on standards that ensure accuracy and compliance. Without them, it's easy to take wrong turns that lead to inaccuracies, rejections, or even audits. Following guidelines also builds a reputation for reliability and accuracy, which is valuable whether you're working independently or as part of a team.

Essential Coding Guidelines Explained

There are a lot of coding guidelines, and not every one will apply to every case. However, some are foundational to coding and apply to almost all cases. Here are a few of the key guidelines that you'll encounter most often and why they're important.

1. Excludes 1 and Excludes 2

The Excludes1 and Excludes2 guidelines are essential for selecting the right code when multiple diagnoses or conditions are present.

- **Excludes 1**: This guideline means "never code these conditions together." Think of Excludes1 as an absolute "do not combine." If two conditions fall under an Excludes1 rule, they represent mutually exclusive situations. For example, if a patient has both a congenital heart defect and an acquired heart condition, you might find that one diagnosis excludes the other under Excludes1, meaning you must pick the one that best applies.

  ☐ **Example**: In the ICD-10-CM, "acute bronchitis" (J20) has an Excludes1 note for "chronic bronchitis" (J42). This tells you not to code both acute and chronic bronchitis together, as they are considered mutually exclusive.

- **Excludes 2**: Excludes 2 is a bit more flexible and means "not included here." You can think of it as a prompt to "code another condition if it's present." For example, if a patient has two conditions listed with an Excludes 2 note, it means both conditions can be coded separately.
  - ☐ **Example**: For conditions like "COPD with acute lower respiratory infection" (J44.0), an Excludes2 note may point you to another code if the patient has a specific type of infection, like pneumonia. You can code both conditions if applicable, but only with the correct guidelines.

Takeaway: Always check for Excludes1 and Excludes2 notes, as they help you avoid double-coding errors or missing critical details.

2. "Code Also" and "Use Additional Code"

These guidelines prompt you to look deeper into the patient's condition and to code additional aspects that may impact the diagnosis. They ensure that you're capturing all relevant aspects of a patient's condition.

- **"Code Also"**: This guideline suggests that another code may be necessary, depending on the full scope of the patient's situation. It's not mandatory, but it reminds you to check if additional details apply.
  - ☐ **Example**: For "Alzheimer's disease" (G30), there's a "code also" instruction to report any associated dementia (F02.80 or F02.81). If dementia is documented, it should be coded in addition to the Alzheimer's code.
- **"Use Additional Code"**: This is a stronger prompt, requiring you to add a secondary code if specific details are documented in the patient's chart. Failing to add these details can result in incomplete coding.
  - ☐ **Example**: For bacterial infections, you'll often see "use additional code to identify organism" with a list of possible codes for the specific bacteria involved. If lab results identify the bacteria, you're required to code it, adding crucial specificity to the diagnosis.

Takeaway: "Code Also" and "Use Additional Code" notes are there to ensure you capture all relevant details, especially if they're documented. When you see these notes, pause and make sure you're including all necessary codes.

3. Laterality

Laterality guidelines indicate whether the condition is on the left, right, or both sides of the body. Failing to code laterality can lead to errors that affect care quality and billing accuracy. For conditions that affect paired organs or limbs, laterality is often crucial.

- **Example**: Suppose a patient has "primary osteoarthritis of the right knee." Coding only "primary osteoarthritis" (M19.90) without specifying laterality (M17.11 for right knee) misses important detail. Using the correct code ensures that the patient's condition is accurately documented for future treatments.

Takeaway: When coding conditions that impact specific body parts, always check for laterality options and choose the correct one based on documentation. It's a small detail that makes a big difference.

4. Combination Codes

Combination codes represent two diagnoses in one code. These codes save time and help prevent confusion in cases where two conditions frequently occur together.

- **Example**: For "diabetes with diabetic nephropathy," you'll find a combination code (E11.21) rather than separate codes for diabetes and nephropathy. Using the combination code simplifies the coding process and ensures that both aspects of the patient's condition are accurately captured.

Takeaway: Combination codes are there to streamline coding. Use them whenever possible to avoid double-coding and ensure you're accurately reflecting the patient's condition.

5. Sequencing Guidelines

Sequencing is all about the order in which codes are listed, and it's critical for coding accuracy and reimbursement. Primary diagnosis codes should reflect the main reason for the patient's visit, while secondary codes capture additional conditions.

- **Example**: Suppose a patient is hospitalized primarily for pneumonia but also has diabetes. Pneumonia would be the primary diagnosis, and diabetes would be secondary. Listing these in the correct order ensures that the primary reason for treatment is prioritized in the coding.

Takeaway: Always list the principal diagnosis first, and make sure secondary codes support and add context to the primary diagnosis.

Practical Tips for Using Guidelines Effectively

Learning to work with guidelines can take time, but here are some strategies to help you make the most of them:

1. **Keep Reference Materials Handy**: Whether it's an ICD-10-CM manual, quick-reference charts, or a digital tool, make sure you have access to the guidelines as you code. Even seasoned coders refer back to guidelines often.
2. **Create a Checklist for Common Guidelines**: If you're regularly coding similar cases, make a checklist of essential guidelines for those cases (Excludes1, Code Also, laterality, etc.). This can save time and ensure you don't overlook important details.
3. **Double-Check Exclusions and Inclusions**: Many errors stem from ignoring Excludes1 or Excludes2 notes. Make it a habit to check for exclusions before finalizing your codes, especially when dealing with complex cases.
4. **Consult a Mentor or Experienced Coder**: If you're stuck on how to apply a guideline, don't hesitate to ask someone more experienced. Guideline application is one of those areas where a second opinion can make a big difference.

Wrapping Up: Turning Guidelines into Your Strength

Guidelines may seem like obstacles at first, but they're the backbone of accurate coding. Once you get familiar with these rules, they become less like restrictions and more like tools that give structure and clarity to each case. As you gain experience, following guidelines will become second nature, and your coding confidence will grow.

Remember, every mistake or correction along the way is a step toward understanding. Embrace the guidelines, and don't be afraid to check and double-check as you learn. You're building habits that will make you a stronger, more reliable coder—and that's a skill worth mastering. Keep at it! You're well on your way to coding with clarity and confidence.

Chapter 4

The Unspecified Trap – Avoiding Generic Codes

"Details matter. In coding, as in life, settling for vagueness leads to misunderstandings, missed opportunities, and a failure to tell the full story."

Welcome to the chapter on what I like to call "the Unspecified Trap," where every coder has likely found themselves at one point or another. "Unspecified" codes can feel like a safe option when documentation is sparse, or when we're just not sure which specific code to use. But beware: overusing unspecified codes is like taking a shortcut that often leads to denied claims, frustrated providers, and lost time for everyone involved.

In this chapter, we'll dive into why unspecified codes can be problematic, when it's okay to use them, and how to avoid falling into the habit of generic coding. And, as always, we'll have a few laughs along the way because we all need a sense of humor when navigating coding guidelines!

My "Unspecified" Overload Moment

Let me start with a story that taught me a lasting lesson about the dangers of unspecified codes. Early in my career, I coded a series of outpatient encounters where "unspecified" became my go-to solution. I was dealing with conditions that sounded vague—like abdominal pain without a clear source, or headaches without more detail in the chart. Each time I hit one of these cases, I defaulted to the unspecified code, thinking, "Hey, better safe than sorry, right?"

Fast forward a few weeks, and I got a call from the billing department. They'd received a wave of denials on my claims due to "lack of specificity."

That's when I learned that unspecified codes are like red flags to insurance companies. It was a rookie mistake, and while it stung, it also taught me a valuable lesson: when in doubt, dig a little deeper.

The Pitfalls of Using Unspecified Codes

Unspecified codes exist for a reason, and sometimes they are the right choice. For instance, in emergency cases or when a patient first presents with symptoms that aren't fully diagnosed, an unspecified code might be all you have. However, over-relying on them can cause several issues:

1. **Claim Denials and Delayed Reimbursement**: Many insurance companies reject claims with unspecified codes, especially if they believe there should have been enough information for a more specific code. Denials can slow down reimbursement, impacting revenue and increasing the workload for everyone involved.
2. **Impact on Patient Care**: When documentation and coding are too vague, it can hinder the continuity of patient care. For example, if the patient's file only shows "unspecified pain," future providers may not know where to begin or how to proceed with treatment.
3. **Inaccurate Data Collection**: Unspecified codes contribute to less accurate healthcare data, which impacts everything from research to resource allocation. Healthcare organizations rely on coding data for decision-making, and generic codes dilute the specificity and usefulness of this data.

So, How Do We Avoid the Unspecified Trap?

Falling back on unspecified codes is tempting, especially when time is tight, but with a few practical strategies, you can learn to avoid them and seek out specificity.

1. Read the Entire Documentation Thoroughly

Sometimes, crucial details are tucked away in parts of the chart you might not read right away. Providers often document specific findings in sections like the review of systems or the plan, which might point you toward a more precise code. Taking a few extra minutes to review all sections of the chart can reveal those specifics that transform an unspecified code into an accurate one.

- **Example**: A patient presents with abdominal pain. The initial impression might seem vague, but a closer read of the documentation might reveal "tenderness in the right lower quadrant," hinting at a possible appendix issue. Rather than coding R10.9 (Unspecified abdominal pain), you could code R10.31 (Right lower quadrant pain).

2. Check for Available Diagnostic Tests or Labs

When you're stuck with vague symptoms, look to see if any diagnostic tests or lab results are referenced in the documentation. Lab results, imaging, or other diagnostic studies often provide clues that can guide you to a more specific diagnosis code.

- **Example**: Let's say a patient presents with "respiratory symptoms" and the initial documentation feels vague. But upon further reading, you find that the provider ordered a chest X-ray showing signs of "pneumonia." Instead of using J98.9 (Respiratory disorder, unspecified), you could code J18.9 (Pneumonia, unspecified organism), which is a more accurate representation.

3. Use Query Forms to Request Specificity

If you encounter documentation that doesn't provide the detail needed for accurate coding, don't hesitate to query the provider. Query forms are there for a reason; they allow you to request clarification or additional detail that can lead to more specific coding.

- **Example**: A provider documents "infection." You could use a query form to ask, "Can you specify the type or source of infection (e.g., bacterial, viral, respiratory, urinary)?" This can provide you with enough information to avoid a generic infection code and instead specify the infection's origin.

4. Familiarize Yourself with Specificity Requirements in Common Conditions

Some conditions commonly fall into the unspecified trap, like diabetes, heart disease, and certain types of pain. Understanding the different variations and requirements for these conditions will make it easier to select specific codes.

- **Example**: For diabetes, specificity requires details like type (Type 1 or Type 2), whether it's controlled or uncontrolled, and whether there are complications (like neuropathy or nephropathy). Knowing these common specificity requirements can help you anticipate what information to look for in the documentation.

5. Create a Cheat Sheet for Common "Unspecified" Offenders

If you notice that you're frequently using unspecified codes for the same types of cases, create a cheat sheet for yourself. List out commonly overused unspecified codes, along with questions to consider or details to look for that would point you to a more specific code.

- **Example**: If you frequently code for "unspecified joint pain" (M25.50), add notes to look for specific joint location (knee, hip, shoulder), side (left or right), and any documented chronicity (acute vs. chronic). This will serve as a reminder to look for these details before settling on a generic code.

When It's Okay to Use Unspecified Codes

There are times when an unspecified code is perfectly appropriate. Here are a few situations where an unspecified code might be the right choice:

1. **Initial Encounters**: For new symptoms or initial encounters, it may be appropriate to use unspecified codes, especially if the provider hasn't determined a specific diagnosis.
2. **Lack of Available Detail**: Sometimes, providers genuinely lack the information to be more specific. If the chart is legitimately sparse and you've reviewed all available documentation, an unspecified code might be your only option.

3. **Emergency Situations**: In emergencies, details may not always be complete. If the patient presents with a life-threatening condition and there isn't time to gather full information, unspecified codes can provide a temporary solution.

Quick Tip: Even if you code something as unspecified initially, revisit the chart later when more information might be available. Often, follow-up visits provide the details needed for specificity.

Making Specificity a Habit

Avoiding unspecified codes isn't just about following guidelines; it's about building habits that make specific coding second nature. Here's how to make specificity a natural part of your process:

1. **Train Your Eye for Key Words**: Look for words in documentation that hint at specifics—like acute, chronic, primary, secondary, mild, moderate, or severe. These keywords often give clues that lead to more precise codes.
2. **Treat Every Encounter as a Learning Opportunity**: Each time you catch yourself about to use an unspecified code, treat it as a mini lesson. Ask yourself, "Is there anything else I can check here?" Over time, this reflection will help you build habits that avoid the generic code trap.
3. **Stay Updated on Coding Guidelines**: Coding conventions evolve, and new guidelines often include details on when specificity is required. Make it a habit to review coding updates, especially those addressing common conditions that could fall into the unspecified trap.
4. **Celebrate Small Wins**: Each time you select a specific code over a generic one, take a moment to recognize your success. It might seem small, but these moments build confidence and reinforce the habit of coding accurately.

Wrapping Up: Avoiding the Unspecified Trap

Mastering the art of specificity in coding takes time, patience, and practice. Remember, using unspecified codes isn't wrong when it's truly necessary, but it's easy to overuse them when you're feeling unsure or short on time. By developing habits that help you seek out specifics, you'll become a more skilled coder, reduce claim denials, and contribute to clearer patient records.

The next time you find yourself about to click on an unspecified code, take a deep breath, review the documentation one more time, and see if there's a way to narrow it down. You're building skills that will serve you for a long time to come, and each effort to add specificity is a win. Keep up the great work—you're well on your way to mastering the art of precision coding!

Chapter 5

Modifier Mayhem – Misunderstanding Modifiers

"Modifiers are the art in the science of coding.

They add nuance, clarity, and depth—when used correctly.

Misused, they muddle the message."

Modifiers are the seasoning in medical coding—they add the special details that tell the full story of a service or procedure. But as essential as they are, modifiers can also be a source of serious headaches. One small modifier mix-up can lead to denied claims, inaccurate billing, or even compliance issues.

In this chapter, we'll dive into the wild world of modifiers, why they're important, and how to avoid common modifier mistakes. Let's start with a story of a modifier misadventure that might sound all too familiar.

My First Modifier Mishap

In my early coding days, I remember dealing with a particularly complex case that involved multiple procedures on the same day. I was feeling confident, thinking I had coded everything correctly, and sent it off. A few weeks later, my manager called me in with a denial report. Turns out, I'd missed a key modifier—one that would have indicated that one of the procedures was distinct from another performed that day. Without that modifier, the insurance saw my coding as a duplicate, resulting in a denial.

That experience taught me that modifiers aren't just "add-ons"; they're critical information that can make or break a claim. Modifiers might seem small, but they can change the whole meaning of a code. From that point on, I learned to treat each modifier like an essential piece of the coding puzzle.

Now, let's walk through the most commonly misused modifiers, with some practical examples to help you understand them better.

Why Modifiers Matter

Modifiers are two-digit codes that provide extra information about a procedure, service, or circumstance that can't be captured with just a primary code. They help clarify details like whether a procedure was done on the left or right side, if it was repeated, or if multiple procedures were distinct from one another. Proper use of modifiers ensures that services are accurately represented and helps prevent denials or delays in reimbursement.

But with dozens of modifiers available, it's easy to see how they can become a source of confusion.

Let's break down some of the most commonly misused modifiers and how to apply them correctly.

Modifier Breakdown: The Most Commonly Misused Modifiers

1. Modifier 25 – "Significant, Separately Identifiable E/M Service"

Modifier 25 is one of the most misunderstood modifiers out there. This modifier is used to indicate that a patient received a significant, separately identifiable evaluation and management (E/M) service on the same day as another procedure. It tells the payer, "Yes, there was an E/M service that wasn't part of the procedure and warrants separate payment."

- **Example**: A patient comes in for a scheduled minor procedure, like a skin lesion removal, but during the visit, they also discuss unrelated symptoms, such as persistent headaches. The provider performs a separate evaluation to assess the headaches. Here, you would attach Modifier 25 to the E/M code to show that the evaluation for the headache was distinct from the lesion removal.
- **Common Mistake**: A common error with Modifier 25 is applying it whenever an E/M service and a procedure occur on the same day, even if the E/M service is directly related to the procedure (for example, checking vitals before the procedure). Modifier 25 should

only be used when the E/M service is significant and separate from the procedure itself.

Takeaway: Use Modifier 25 only when the E/M service is truly distinct from any other procedure provided that day. Look for documentation that supports a separate and unrelated assessment.

2. Modifier 59 – "Distinct Procedural Service"

Modifier 59 is used to indicate that two procedures are distinct and separate from each other, even if they were performed on the same day. This is often necessary when two codes might otherwise seem like duplicates to payers. Modifier 59 clarifies that each procedure addressed a different problem or was performed on a different body area.

- **Example**: Suppose a patient has two procedures on the same day—one for removing a foreign body from the right hand and another for the left hand. Here, Modifier 59 would be used with one of the procedure codes to indicate that each procedure was distinct and performed on different sites.
- **Common Mistake**: Modifier 59 is frequently overused to bypass edits, which can lead to compliance issues. Avoid using it just to push a claim through without verifying that the procedures truly meet the criteria for "distinct and separate."

Takeaway: Use Modifier 59 only when the documentation supports that the procedures were separate and unrelated. Modifier 59 is one of the most scrutinized modifiers, so only apply it when it's absolutely justified.

3. Modifier 51 – "Multiple Procedures"

Modifier 51 is applied when multiple procedures are performed during the same session. This tells payers that multiple services were provided and allows them to apply any reductions or adjustments based on that.

- **Example**: A patient undergoes both a tonsillectomy and adenoidectomy during the same operative session. You would use Modifier 51 with the secondary procedure to indicate that both procedures were performed together.
- **Common Mistake**: Some coders apply Modifier 51 to all procedures performed on the same day, even those with modifier codes that

inherently indicate multiple procedures (like Modifier 59). Modifier 51 should only be used on additional procedures that meet the criteria of being performed in the same session and that don't have specific modifiers indicating a distinct or separate service.

Takeaway: Use Modifier 51 only when multiple procedures meet the criteria for the same session. Avoid stacking it with other modifiers, like 59, as they serve different purposes.

4. Modifier 76 – "Repeat Procedure by Same Physician"

Modifier 76 is used when a provider repeats a procedure on the same day for the same patient. This modifier signals that the procedure was legitimately repeated, rather than being mistakenly duplicated.

- **Example**: A patient has a diagnostic EKG in the morning, and then later that same day, they undergo another EKG due to changes in their symptoms. You'd attach Modifier 76 to the second EKG code to show that the repeat test was medically necessary.
- **Common Mistake**: Modifier 76 is sometimes used when a different provider repeats the procedure, which would actually require Modifier 77 (repeat procedure by another provider). Modifier 76 should only be used when the same provider repeats the procedure.

Takeaway: Use Modifier 76 only for procedures repeated by the same provider on the same day. For repeat procedures by different providers, use Modifier 77 instead.

5. Modifier 24 – "Unrelated E/M Service by the Same Physician During a Postoperative Period"

Modifier 24 is essential when a patient is seen for an unrelated E/M service during the global period of a previous surgery. This modifier helps clarify that the E/M service provided has nothing to do with the post-op care for the surgery and should be reimbursed separately.

- **Example**: A patient has knee surgery and returns during the global period for an unrelated issue, such as a skin rash. Modifier 24 would be used with the E/M code for the skin rash visit to show that this visit was unrelated to the surgery.

- **Common Mistake**: Applying Modifier 24 to any E/M service during a global period, even if it relates to the surgical recovery. Modifier 24 should only be used for conditions that are truly unrelated to the surgery.

Takeaway: Only use Modifier 24 when the E/M service is for an issue completely unrelated to the recent surgery. The documentation should clearly support that it's unrelated.

Tips for Avoiding Modifier Mayhem

1. **Review Documentation Carefully**: Modifiers rely heavily on documentation. Make sure the provider's notes support the use of the modifier and that it's clear why the service is distinct, separate, or otherwise modified.
2. **Use a Modifier Decision Tree**: Some practices use modifier decision trees or flowcharts to help coders make consistent decisions about when to apply modifiers. This can be especially helpful when you're new to coding or facing complex cases.
3. **Stay Updated on Payer Guidelines**: Different payers sometimes have specific rules for modifier use. If you frequently code for a particular payer, familiarize yourself with their modifier guidelines to avoid denials.
4. **Practice with Common Scenarios**: Practicing with example cases that include multiple services or complex procedures can help you become more confident in using modifiers accurately. Over time, these decisions will become second nature.
5. **Don't Overuse "Just in Case"**: It can be tempting to throw in a modifier "just in case" you missed something. However, improper use of modifiers is a red flag to payers. Only apply modifiers when the documentation and circumstances clearly support it.

Wrapping Up: Mastering Modifier Use

Modifiers add depth and accuracy to coding, allowing the full picture of a patient's care to come through. They're like the punctuation in a sentence—small but essential to getting the meaning right. As you get more comfortable with modifiers, you'll find they aren't so much a source of "mayhem" as a helpful tool for making sure every procedure and service is represented accurately.

Remember, everyone stumbles with modifiers at some point. Each time you use one, take a moment to check the documentation and ensure it's appropriate. With a little extra care, you'll be coding with confidence, and modifiers will feel less like mayhem and more like second nature.

Keep going! You're building expertise with each code you choose, and mastering modifiers is just one more step on your journey to coding confidence.

Chapter 6

Audit Anxiety – Facing and Learning from Audits

"An audit is not a judgment—it's a mirror that reflects your work, your growth, and the areas that still need polishing."

Audits are a part of every coder's life, and just the thought of one can bring on a little wave of nervousness. When it's an external audit—a review by auditors outside your own organization—the pressure can feel even higher. But here's the thing: audits are not just about finding errors; they're about ensuring accuracy, refining skills, and ultimately helping us become better coders.

In this chapter, we'll dive into ways to turn audit anxiety into a growth opportunity. I'll share a story from my first experience with an external audit—a moment that turned out to be more beneficial than I expected—and provide practical steps to help you approach audits with confidence.

My First External Audit Story

One day, I logged in to find an email marked "External Audit Notification" waiting for me. My stomach did a flip as I read that an external auditor would be reviewing a selection of charts I had coded a few months back. My heart raced as I read the details: the cases they'd selected included a particularly complex one involving multiple procedures, some tricky modifiers, and specific diagnostic codes. I remembered the case well, and suddenly, I began to second-guess every choice I'd made.

When the audit results finally came back, they'd flagged a couple of issues. One was a modifier error where I'd used one modifier when another was required, and the other was a missed opportunity to be more specific with a diagnosis code. Seeing the corrections wasn't easy, but it was helpful. That audit taught me a lot about precision, particularly when it came to modifiers and specificity, and I realized that an external audit could be one of the best opportunities to learn and improve.

Why External Audits Happen (And Why They're a Good Thing)

External audits happen for a variety of reasons: as part of routine compliance checks, for quality assurance, or sometimes as a targeted review when an organization wants to ensure accuracy. The purpose of these audits isn't to "catch" coders but to maintain high standards, improve reimbursement accuracy, and support patient care by ensuring the information is precise and complete.

Think of an external audit as an opportunity to get feedback from experienced reviewers. It's normal to feel a little apprehensive, but by approaching it with an open mind, an audit can provide insights that help you grow as a coder.

How to Prepare for an External Audit Without Breaking a Sweat

Being prepared can make all the difference when it comes to an audit. Here's a step-by-step guide to help you prepare, so you can feel calm and ready when the time comes.

1. Organize Your Documentation

Clear and organized documentation is essential during an audit. Every coding choice should be supported by the clinical documentation in the file, and any additional notes should be easily accessible.

- **Tip**: Make it a habit to add brief notes explaining complex coding decisions, especially when working with difficult cases. A short note about why you selected a specific code or modifier can be incredibly helpful if that case is ever audited.

2. Stay Updated on Coding Guidelines and Changes

Guidelines and standards change frequently, and audits often catch areas where coders may be using outdated practices. Set aside a little time each week to review any updates in coding standards or payer-specific guidelines to stay current.

- **Example**: If you see new guidance about a particular modifier, update any personal reference notes you keep. Staying updated helps prevent misunderstandings that can lead to audit findings.

3. Double-Check Common Problem Areas

Certain coding areas, like modifiers, unspecified codes, and procedure bundling, are more frequently scrutinized during audits. Double-checking these areas can help prevent common errors.

- **Modifier Mistakes**: Modifiers are frequently reviewed during audits, so make sure every modifier has a clear purpose backed by documentation. Misused modifiers are often flagged in audits, so double-check them whenever you use one.
- **Unspecified Codes**: Auditors expect specificity in coding whenever possible, so avoid unspecified codes if the documentation supports something more specific.

4. Keep a Personal "Audit Log" of Key Learning Points

Each audit is a chance to learn something new. Create a personal "audit log" where you track common findings or issues that auditors have flagged in the past. This log can serve as a reminder to watch out for similar issues in future coding.

- **Example**: If an audit once flagged an issue with a particular modifier, note it in your audit log as a reminder to review modifiers carefully in similar cases. Over time, this log will become a valuable reference to prevent repeat findings.

Staying Calm and Confident During an External Audit

When you know an audit is happening, it's natural to feel a bit of anxiety. Here's how to approach the process with confidence, turning it into a productive experience.

1. Trust Your Training and Experience

Remember that you've put in the work to become a skilled coder, and an audit doesn't change that. Audits are simply there to ensure standards are met. Trust in your training and experience, and approach the audit as a normal part of your professional life.

2. See the Auditor as a Resource, Not a Critic

External auditors are there to help uphold quality standards. Rather than viewing them as critics, approach them as resources who can provide valuable insight.

- **Example**: If you're unclear why an auditor flagged a particular issue, ask for clarification. Understanding their perspective helps you apply best practices and learn from the process.

3. Focus on Learning, Not Perfection

Expecting perfection during an audit can lead to unnecessary stress. Approach audits with a mindset of learning rather than perfection. Coding is complex, and everyone makes mistakes. Use each audit as a learning tool to improve.

- **Tip**: Remind yourself that even experienced coders face corrections. Each audit is a checkpoint that helps you refine your skills, not a judgment of your abilities.

Learning from Audit Findings

Audits are goldmines for personal growth. Each finding is a chance to understand something new about coding. Here's how to turn audit feedback into a powerful tool for improvement.

1. Review Findings with an Open Mind

When you receive feedback, approach it without getting defensive. Ask yourself, "What can I learn from this?" Each finding is an opportunity to improve.

- **Example**: If an auditor points out that you could have used a specific code instead of a generic one, take it as a reminder to prioritize specificity in the future. These adjustments become second nature over time.

2. Incorporate Feedback into Your Routine

One of the best ways to learn from audit feedback is to build corrective actions into your daily routine. If you're often flagged for a particular issue, give it extra attention in future cases.

- **Example**: If you've been corrected on modifier use, add a "modifier review" step into your coding checklist to make sure you're consistently applying them correctly. These routines will reinforce good habits and prevent future errors.

3. Track Your Progress

Audits give you a chance to measure improvement over time. As you go through more audits, compare findings to see how far you've come.

- **Tip**: Celebrate improvements, even if they're small. Coding accuracy builds over time, and every positive audit result is a sign of progress worth acknowledging.

Preparing for Future External Audits

Since external audits can come from a variety of sources, being proactive is essential. Here are a few additional tips to keep in mind:

1. **Ensure Documentation Is Accessible and Complete**: External auditors rely on complete and clear documentation to verify coding. Make sure every case is well-documented and organized.
2. **Stay in Communication with Your Team**: External audits may involve departments beyond coding, like billing or compliance. Communicate openly to make sure everyone involved has the necessary information and support.
3. **Proactively Address Findings from Past Audits**: If you've had audit findings in the past, proactively address those areas in future cases. Demonstrating improvement in these areas shows auditors that you're dedicated to accuracy.

Wrapping Up: Turning External Audit Anxiety into Coding Confidence

External audits may feel daunting, but they're a natural part of the coding profession and an essential tool for upholding high standards. By approaching each audit with a positive mindset, being prepared, and viewing auditors as resources, you can transform audit anxiety into confidence.

Remember, no coder is perfect, and every audit is a chance to learn and grow. With the right perspective, you can use audits as valuable checkpoints on your journey to becoming a skilled and knowledgeable coder. So, the next time you receive that audit notification, take a deep breath, trust your work, and look forward to another step in your path to mastery.

You're building a skill set that only grows stronger with experience. Keep coding confidently—you're well on your way!

Chapter 7

The Denial Dance – Tackling Denials and Rejections

"Every denial is a chance to rewrite the story. Instead of frustration, see it as an invitation to improve, to clarify, and to try again."

Denials are a part of every coder's journey. Just when you think you've nailed down the details, a denial notification pops up, leaving you scratching your head. Few things are as frustrating as seeing the work you spent hours on get rejected. But here's the good news: denials are some of the best opportunities to learn, refine your skills, and navigate the complex world of healthcare reimbursement.

In this chapter, we'll dive into some common reasons for denials, strategies to prevent them, and effective steps for handling them when they happen. Let's start with a story about one of my earliest denials—a case I still remember well—because it taught me a few lessons I still carry with me today.

The Case That Taught Me to Dance Through Denials

Early in my career, I was tasked with coding a complex outpatient surgery case. The patient had come in for an arthroscopy with debridement and repair of a torn meniscus. It was a multi-step procedure, with additional details about specific locations and complexities in the knee, so I'd been meticulous about capturing every aspect. The case involved:

- **Arthroscopy**: Viewing the inside of the knee with a tiny camera.
- **Debridement**: Cleaning out damaged tissue.

- **Meniscal Repair**: Repairing the torn section of the meniscus, with distinct work done on the lateral portion and some touch-ups on the medial section.

I'd carefully applied codes for each part, added modifiers to account for different areas worked on, and double-checked the documentation to make sure I wasn't missing anything. Feeling confident, I submitted it and moved on.

A few weeks later, a denial notification landed in my inbox: "Claim denied for incorrect modifier usage." I was baffled. I'd used Modifier 59 to indicate that the meniscal repair was separate from the debridement. But after reviewing the explanation of benefits (EOB) and digging into payer guidelines, I discovered that I should have used Modifier XS instead of Modifier 59, as the payer required this modifier for services in "distinct procedural services in separate structures."

That small oversight—using Modifier 59 when the payer preferred Modifier XS—caused the entire claim to be denied. It was a hard lesson, but one that taught me the importance of knowing each payer's preferences and double-checking modifier usage before submission. Now, let's explore the most common reasons for denials and how to handle them, so you can turn these experiences into growth opportunities.

Common Reasons for Denials (And How to Avoid Them)

Understanding the common reasons for denials is the first step to reducing their occurrence. Here are the main culprits and practical ways to prevent them.

1. Incorrect or Missing Modifiers

Modifiers are the small but powerful details that clarify a procedure, such as whether it was done on the left or right side, was distinct from another procedure, or involved multiple sessions. Modifiers help paint a clear picture of services, but using the wrong one can lead to denials.

- **Prevention Tip**: Familiarize yourself with commonly used modifiers and check payer guidelines for preferences, like XS versus 59.

Double-check all modifiers before submitting claims, especially in multi-procedure cases.

- **Example**: If you're coding for procedures on different structures, like in the knee case I encountered, use Modifier XS instead of 59 if the payer specifies. It's a subtle difference, but it ensures compliance with payer preferences.

2. Lack of Specificity in Diagnosis Codes

Using unspecified codes when a more specific code exists can lead to denials, as payers expect details that accurately reflect the patient's condition. Coding "abdominal pain, unspecified" when the notes specify "right lower quadrant abdominal pain" could lead to a denial.

- **Prevention Tip**: Use the most specific diagnosis code available based on documentation. If the documentation provides specifics about location, severity, or chronicity, make sure the code captures that level of detail.
- **Example**: If a patient presents with "chronic, right-sided knee pain," make sure to select a code that includes both "chronic" and "right side" instead of a generic "knee pain" code.

3. Insufficient Documentation

Denials often happen because the documentation doesn't fully support the codes used. If key details are missing, such as laterality, procedural notes, or the medical necessity of a service, payers may deny the claim.

- **Prevention Tip**: Make sure the documentation is thorough and covers all necessary details for accurate coding. For surgical procedures, ensure the provider has documented the reason, specific steps, and any unique circumstances that impact coding.
- **Example**: In a case where multiple parts of a knee are treated, ensure that the documentation specifies each area and procedure performed. A clear breakdown helps avoid confusion and unnecessary denials.

4. Non-Covered Services or Outdated Codes

Claims can be denied if the service isn't covered under the patient's plan or if an outdated code is used. Some services have specific coverage requirements, and coding standards frequently change.

- **Prevention Tip**: Verify the coverage policy for the service and make sure all codes are current. Set aside time to review coding updates and payer-specific policies regularly. If a service requires prior authorization, confirm that it's been approved.
- **Example**: For a preventive procedure, check if the patient's plan includes coverage for preventive services. Some plans cover preventive services fully, while others have restrictions.

5. Duplicate Claims or Incorrect Bundling

When services that should be bundled are billed separately, or when a claim is mistakenly resubmitted, denials for duplicates or incorrect submissions often follow. For example, billing separately for two components of a bundled procedure will likely trigger a denial.

- **Prevention Tip**: Use resources like the Correct Coding Initiative (CCI) edits to verify correct bundling and avoid submitting duplicate claims. If a duplicate submission is necessary, make sure to include notes explaining why.
- **Example**: When a patient has a comprehensive exam and a minor procedure on the same day, check if these services are bundled before billing separately. If CCI edits indicate bundling, apply the appropriate bundled code.

Steps for Handling a Denial

Denials happen, but having a structured approach can turn them from setbacks into solutions. Here's how to tackle a denial step-by-step.

1. Identify the Denial Reason

Start by carefully reviewing the Explanation of Benefits (EOB) or Remittance Advice (RA) to determine the exact reason for the denial. These documents provide codes and explanations that can help you pinpoint where things went wrong.

- **Example**: If the denial reason is "incorrect modifier," go back to the documentation and identify where an alternate modifier (like XS versus 59) should have been used.

2. Gather All Relevant Documentation

Once you know why the claim was denied, gather any supporting documentation for the case. This is essential, especially if you need to appeal the denial. If the denial was due to lack of specificity, for example, check for any additional details in the patient's record.

- **Example**: For a surgical procedure denied due to "insufficient documentation," locate the operative notes and any follow-up records that explain the necessity and details of the procedure.

3. Determine Whether a Correction or Appeal Is Needed

Some denials can be fixed with a simple correction, while others may require a formal appeal. If the issue is straightforward, like a missing modifier, a correction may be enough. But if the issue involves medical necessity or coding specificity, a more detailed appeal may be required.

- **Correction Example**: If the denial is due to a missing modifier, add the correct modifier and resubmit.
- **Appeal Example**: For a denial citing "lack of medical necessity," gather relevant clinical notes that explain the necessity and submit an appeal with a detailed explanation.

4. Submit the Correction or Appeal Promptly

Most payers have strict timelines for submitting appeals or corrections. Delays can result in missed appeal deadlines, so it's essential to submit any corrections or appeals promptly. Include all necessary supporting documentation.

- **Tip**: Create a checklist for necessary documents before submission to ensure everything is included, which can help avoid further delays.

5. Track the Outcome and Document Lessons Learned

Once the denial is resolved, make a note of the reason and the solution. Keeping a record of these cases helps you identify patterns, build your knowledge, and avoid similar issues in the future.

- **Example**: If you notice a pattern of denials related to modifier use, add a modifier review step to your pre-submission routine.

Turning Denial Frustration into Growth

Denials can be frustrating, but they're also valuable learning tools. By tracking denial reasons and identifying patterns, you can continuously improve your coding process and prevent similar issues in the future. Here's how to make each denial a learning opportunity.

1. **Keep a Denial Log**: Record each denial, its reason, and how it was resolved. This log becomes a powerful resource for spotting common issues and reinforcing accurate coding practices.
2. **Treat Denials as Case Studies**: Take time to analyze each denial as a case study. Break down the issue, review how it was resolved, and note any lessons learned. This process will turn each denial into a practical learning experience.
3. **Implement Preventive Routines**: Set up checklists or routines to catch recurring issues before they lead to denials. For instance, if denials for specificity are common, add a final "specificity check" to your process before submission.
4. **Celebrate Wins**: Successfully resolving a denial, or seeing a reduction in denials over time, is worth celebrating. These victories build your confidence and reinforce good habits, turning denials into milestones in your professional growth.

Wrapping Up: Dancing Through Denials

The "denial dance" is a normal part of coding, and while it can be frustrating, each denial also offers a chance to grow. By understanding common reasons for denials, developing a structured approach for addressing them, and learning from each experience, you'll not only reduce your denial rate but also become a more skilled coder.

Remember, denials aren't a reflection of your abilities—they're simply part of the process. With the right approach, every denial can become a step in your journey to coding mastery. So, the next time a denial comes your way, take a deep breath, dive into the details, and treat it as one more opportunity to refine your skills.

You've got this, and every denial you handle gets you closer to becoming a coding pro!

Chapter 8

Ethics Under Pressure – Navigating Gray Areas in Coding

"Integrity is what you do when no one is watching. In coding, every choice reflects your commitment to doing the right thing—even when it's hard."

Working as a medical coder in an outsourced setting brings unique challenges, especially when it comes to maintaining ethical standards. When handling coding for external clients, there may be subtle or direct pressures to code in ways that maximize reimbursement or align with specific business goals, even if that conflicts with coding guidelines. These moments put our integrity to the test, especially when dealing with high-stakes cases where minor code changes could make a big financial difference.

In this chapter, we'll discuss the importance of ethical coding and how to handle real-world situations that push ethical boundaries. Let's start with a story that highlights one such dilemma, a scenario that taught me early on that ethics are foundational to our work in coding.

The Temptation to "Enhance" a Code

A few years back, my team and I were working on a high-profile project coding orthopedic cases. Our client, a large healthcare provider, was focused on improving reimbursement for specific surgical procedures and closely tracked our coding submissions. For one particular project, we were working on complex spinal surgeries where the potential for higher reimbursement was significant if codes reflected the maximum level of involvement and complexity.

One day, I was reviewing a spinal fusion case—a procedure to connect two or more vertebrae. The documentation included notes on additional bone grafts and fusion to multiple segments of the spine. However, the exact number of vertebral levels involved wasn't clearly detailed in the operative report. To accurately code it, we needed to know the number of segments, which directly impacts coding complexity and reimbursement.

When I reached out to our team lead for clarification, the response came back from the client's representative: "Let's assume it was the maximum number of levels, considering the usual approach for this surgeon." In other words, the client was suggesting that we code for a higher level of complexity than what the documentation supported. The pressure was clear: the client wanted the highest code possible, even if it meant interpreting the documentation in their favor.

After considering it carefully, I decided to flag the case back, explaining that we couldn't assume complexity without explicit documentation of the number of levels involved. Instead, I suggested requesting additional clarification from the provider to ensure the coding was accurate. It wasn't the answer the client wanted, but sticking to this decision meant upholding the accuracy and ethics required in coding.

Why Ethical Standards Are Essential in Medical Coding

Accurate and ethical coding does more than ensure fair payment; it also safeguards patient records, compliance, and the integrity of healthcare data. Here's why ethical coding matters:

1. **Patient Care**: Coding directly impacts patient records. Overstated complexity or added procedures that weren't documented can distort a patient's medical history, affecting their future care.
2. **Fair Reimbursement**: Accurate coding ensures fair reimbursement based on services actually provided. Overstated codes can lead to inflated billing, audits, and potential legal issues.
3. **Legal Compliance**: Coding must align with payer guidelines and government regulations to avoid penalties or legal action. Unethical coding practices put the organization—and the coders involved—at risk.

Navigating Common Ethical Gray Areas in Coding

Handling ethical challenges requires confidence in coding guidelines and a commitment to integrity. Let's look at some common ethical gray areas and how to respond to them effectively.

1. Pressure to Assume or "Enhance" Code Complexity

Clients sometimes encourage coders to "assume" the maximum level of complexity or add modifiers that suggest higher involvement than documentation supports. This can be tempting, especially when the pressure to maximize reimbursement is high.

- **How to Handle It**: Stick with the documentation and ask for clarification if details are missing. Politely explain that codes must directly reflect documented information. If the complexity isn't clear, request additional documentation rather than making assumptions.
- **Example**: If you're coding a multi-level spinal fusion and the documentation doesn't specify the number of levels, don't assume the highest complexity. Explain that the missing details prevent accurate coding and request clarification from the provider if possible.

2. Requests to Split Codes for Higher Reimbursement

In some cases, clients may suggest splitting bundled services to code separately for each, even if they should be combined. For example, certain procedures are considered comprehensive, with smaller services bundled within them. Unbundling can lead to denials or compliance issues.

- **How to Handle It**: Follow the National Correct Coding Initiative (NCCI) guidelines and apply bundled codes when applicable. If a client questions why services are bundled, reference NCCI rules and explain that these guidelines are standard for accurate and compliant coding.
- **Example**: Suppose you're coding for a surgical procedure that includes both an incision and closure, but the client suggests coding the incision separately to increase reimbursement. Explain that NCCI guidelines require that these services be bundled and that billing them separately would go against compliance standards.

3. Pressure to Add Secondary Diagnoses or Conditions

Clients may encourage coders to add secondary diagnoses, complications, or comorbidities to justify a higher level of care, even if these conditions aren't directly documented or relevant to the primary service. This can create an inflated picture of the patient's condition.

- **How to Handle It**: Only code for diagnoses or conditions that are documented as relevant to the encounter. Explain that coding must accurately reflect the documented encounter and that secondary conditions should only be coded if they're directly addressed or impact the treatment provided.
- **Example**: Imagine you're coding for a patient's knee replacement surgery, and the client suggests adding a secondary diagnosis like hypertension to highlight the case's complexity. Before including it, check the documentation:
    - Was hypertension addressed during the encounter (e.g., medication adjustment, blood pressure monitoring)?
    - Did it influence the treatment plan or surgical approach?

If there's no documentation indicating that hypertension impacted the care provided or was actively managed, it's inappropriate to code it. Coding hypertension in this case would misrepresent the patient's clinical scenario and violate compliance guidelines.

4. Encouragement to Use "Ambiguous" Codes When Specific Codes Exist

In some cases, clients may suggest using vague or non-specific codes, thinking it will make the coding process easier or avoid scrutiny. This practice, however, can lead to inaccurate records and potential denials.

- **How to Handle It**: Always select the most specific code that aligns with the documentation. Explain that specificity in coding not only prevents denials but also ensures accurate records, which support patient care and compliance.
- **Example**: If a provider documents "acute bronchitis," but the client suggests coding it under a more general respiratory condition, explain that accurate coding should reflect the specific diagnosis to avoid denials and support future patient care.

Responding to Ethical Pressure with Professionalism

Handling ethical pressure doesn't have to be confrontational. Here are strategies to respond professionally while upholding your ethical standards.

1. **Reference Guidelines**: When asked to bend rules, politely refer to coding standards, guidelines, or NCCI edits that support your decision. Using guidelines as your basis keeps the conversation professional and grounded in established rules.
2. **Suggest Requesting Documentation Updates**: If the client pushes for a code that isn't documented, suggest that they request an update from the provider. This keeps your coding aligned with the documentation and offers a solution that maintains accuracy.
3. **Seek Support from Supervisors**: If you're ever unsure or feel pressured to code unethically, bring the issue to a supervisor or compliance officer. They can offer guidance, reinforce your decision, or communicate directly with the client if needed.
4. **Document Your Concerns**: Keep a record of any situations where you feel pressured to code unethically. Documenting your concerns provides a record that protects you if there's ever a question about your coding decisions.

Building an Ethical Coding Routine

Developing habits that reinforce ethical coding practices can help you avoid gray areas and build a reputation for integrity. Here's how to establish an ethical coding routine:

1. **Double-Check Documentation**: Make it a habit to cross-check documentation with the codes you select. When in doubt, request clarification rather than making assumptions.
2. **Stay Informed on Coding Standards**: Keeping up-to-date with guidelines, NCCI edits, and payer-specific rules ensures you have the information needed to make accurate and compliant coding decisions.

3. **Prioritize Integrity Over Speed**: Ethical coding may take a little longer, especially when cases are complex, but accuracy and integrity are always worth the extra time. Avoid rushing through codes, particularly in cases with financial pressure.
4. **Reflect on Ethical Scenarios**: Consider potential gray areas and practice responding to them so that, when faced with real situations, you feel confident handling them ethically.

Wrapping Up: Ethics as the Foundation of Coding

In coding, ethical choices impact everything from patient care to compliance and reimbursement. When faced with pressures to "enhance" codes, split bundles, or add unsubstantiated conditions, remember that your responsibility is to represent each case truthfully. Standing by your ethical standards isn't just about following rules; it's about protecting patient records, upholding compliance, and maintaining your own integrity.

The next time you're faced with an ethical gray area, remember that choosing accuracy is choosing honesty—and that decision will always be worth it. You're building a foundation of integrity that will serve you throughout your career in coding. Keep up the great work; your commitment to ethics strengthens the field of medical coding and sets a high standard for everyone around you.

Chapter 9

The Reimbursement Roadmap – Following the Money

"Behind every dollar is a decision, and behind every decision is a story. Understand the flow of reimbursement, and you'll see the full picture."

Medical coding isn't just about selecting the correct codes; it's also about understanding how those codes impact the financial side of healthcare. Every code we assign directly affects the reimbursement a provider receives, which in turn impacts the sustainability of the healthcare organization, its ability to serve patients, and its resources for future care. Coders, in a real sense, help steer the "reimbursement roadmap" for healthcare.

In this chapter, we'll break down the reimbursement process, explore the impact of coding accuracy on financial outcomes, and walk through the cycle of how a claim goes from submission to payment. Let's start with a story that shows just how powerful accurate coding can be in the world of healthcare finance.

A Lesson in Financial Impact: The Case of the "Lost Modifier"

Early in my career, I was working on a batch of claims for orthopedic surgeries. One particular case involved a complicated hip replacement procedure. I coded it according to the documentation but missed a key modifier that signified the procedure was bilateral—performed on both sides, not just one. Since the modifier was missing, the claim processed as if the surgeon had only operated on one side, reducing the reimbursement by nearly half.

A few weeks later, I received a notice from the billing department: the claim had underpaid, and they needed to investigate why. When they pulled up the claim details, they noticed the missing modifier. Correcting it and resubmitting the claim took extra time, and because of the error, the organization faced delays in receiving full payment.

This experience taught me how closely coding accuracy is tied to financial outcomes. A single modifier affected thousands of dollars and added to the workload of multiple departments. From that day forward, I developed a checklist for modifiers on complex procedures, ensuring every code I submitted was as complete and accurate as possible. This was my first real encounter with the financial impact of coding and a reminder that every detail matters.

The Reimbursement Cycle: How Coding Fits In

The reimbursement cycle, sometimes called the revenue cycle, is a multi-step process that involves coding, billing, claims submission, and payment. Coders play a foundational role in this cycle by ensuring that each procedure and diagnosis is coded accurately, which forms the basis for claim submissions. Here's a breakdown of the reimbursement cycle and how each step connects back to coding.

1. Patient Encounter and Documentation

The reimbursement cycle begins when a patient receives care. After the encounter, the healthcare provider documents the services rendered, including diagnoses, procedures, and any relevant clinical details. This documentation is critical, as it forms the basis for coding.

- **Impact of Coding**: Accurate and complete documentation allows coders to choose the correct codes. If documentation is vague or incomplete, it can lead to coding errors, which may cause denials or delayed payments later in the cycle.

2. Coding for Diagnosis and Procedures

Next, coders review the documentation to assign diagnosis codes (ICD-10-CM), procedure codes (CPT or HCPCS), and any necessary modifiers. This step is crucial, as the codes determine the type and level of reimbursement the provider will receive.

- **Impact of Coding**: Codes must be both accurate and specific to avoid denials. For example, using a general code for a specific condition may result in underpayment, while overcoding can lead to audits and financial penalties.

3. Claims Submission

Once coding is complete, the billing team creates a claim that includes all relevant codes, modifiers, and patient information. This claim is then submitted to the insurance company or payer for review and reimbursement.

- **Impact of Coding**: The codes submitted on the claim directly affect how the payer processes the claim. Inaccurate or incomplete coding can trigger payer edits that result in claim rejections or delays, slowing down the entire reimbursement cycle.

4. Payer Review and Adjudication

After receiving the claim, the payer reviews it to ensure compliance with coverage policies, coding guidelines, and contractual agreements. The payer then either approves, denies, or adjusts the claim based on the information provided.

- **Impact of Coding**: Accurate coding minimizes the likelihood of denials and adjustments. If a payer identifies issues such as upcoding, missing modifiers, or unspecified codes, they may reduce reimbursement or deny the claim outright.

5. Payment and Reconciliation

If the claim is approved, the payer issues payment to the provider. This payment is then reconciled with the initial claim to ensure accuracy. Any discrepancies may lead to additional review or adjustments.

- **Impact of Coding**: Proper coding ensures that the payment received matches the expected reimbursement for the services provided. Errors at this stage can affect revenue forecasting and budgeting for the healthcare organization.

Common Coding Errors and Their Financial Impact

Let's explore some common coding errors and how they impact the financial aspect of healthcare, including delayed payments, claim denials, and financial compliance risks.

1. Incorrect or Missing Modifiers

Modifiers provide essential details about a procedure, like if it was bilateral, if there were multiple surgeries, or if it was done in a unique setting. Missing or incorrect modifiers often lead to claim rejections or reduced payments.

- **Financial Impact**: Modifiers can drastically change the amount reimbursed. For example, missing a modifier on a bilateral procedure means the claim may only reimburse for one side, potentially cutting reimbursement in half.

2. Unspecified or Inaccurate Diagnosis Codes

Using unspecified diagnosis codes, especially when more specific ones are available, can result in denied claims. Payers expect a high level of specificity to justify the level of care provided.

- **Financial Impact**: Unspecified codes can result in partial payments or denials, affecting the organization's revenue and potentially leading to rework if the claim is resubmitted with more accurate codes.

3. Upcoding or Downcoding

Upcoding (using a higher-paying code than appropriate) and downcoding (using a lower-paying code than required) can cause compliance issues. Upcoding can lead to audits and penalties, while downcoding can result in underpayment.

- **Financial Impact**: Upcoding can bring short-term reimbursement gains, but it poses a high risk for audits, repayments, and fines. Downcoding, on the other hand, reduces revenue and can hinder the organization's financial stability.

4. Errors in Procedure Bundling

Procedure bundling guidelines, like those from the National Correct Coding Initiative (NCCI), dictate when procedures should be billed together. Failing to follow these guidelines can lead to claim denials and compliance issues.

- **Financial Impact**: Errors in bundling may result in denied claims, requiring resubmission or adjustments that delay payment. They also risk financial penalties if audits reveal repeated unbundling errors.

Best Practices for Supporting Financial Integrity in Coding

Accuracy in coding is foundational to ensuring that the reimbursement process runs smoothly and fairly. Here are some best practices to help coders support financial integrity.

1. Stay Current on Coding Guidelines

Guidelines change frequently, impacting everything from modifier usage to procedure bundling. Staying current helps you code accurately and avoid issues that lead to denials.

- **Practical Tip**: Set aside time each week to review updates from sources like the American Medical Association (AMA), CMS, or payer-specific bulletins. Keeping up-to-date prevents costly errors.

2. Double-Check High-Impact Cases

For high-stakes procedures, such as surgeries or multi-step treatments, taking extra time to review each code and modifier can make a huge difference in financial outcomes.

- **Practical Tip**: Create a checklist for high-impact cases that includes common issues like laterality, modifiers, and specificity. Double-checking can prevent significant underpayments or denials.

3. Use Specific Codes and Avoid Generalizations

Whenever possible, use specific diagnosis and procedure codes that align closely with documentation. This reduces the likelihood of denials and ensures accurate reimbursement.

- **Practical Tip**: If documentation is unclear, reach out to a supervisor or query the provider to clarify before using unspecified codes. It saves time and ensures that reimbursement is maximized accurately.

4. Track Denials and Identify Patterns

If you encounter frequent denials, keep a log to track the reasons. Identifying patterns in denials can reveal areas where coding practices need adjustment.

- **Practical Tip**: Regularly review your denial log to identify and address recurring issues. It's a proactive way to reduce errors that impact reimbursement.

5. Communicate with Billing and Revenue Cycle Teams

The reimbursement cycle depends on communication between coders, billers, and other revenue cycle staff. Collaborating helps ensure that coding choices align with billing practices and payer expectations.

- **Practical Tip**: Set up regular check-ins with billing teams to review common issues, denial trends, and ways to improve the accuracy of submissions.

The Bigger Picture: Coding's Role in Financial Stability

In coding, we often focus on accuracy for the sake of compliance and quality, but the broader impact of correct coding extends to the financial stability of healthcare organizations. Each claim we code correctly brings in the revenue needed to keep facilities running, pay providers, and maintain patient services.

Moreover, accurate coding contributes to the integrity of healthcare data, which informs policy, resource allocation, and healthcare improvements on a national level. By understanding the role coding plays in the larger financial landscape, coders can see their work as essential to both their organization's success and the overall health of the healthcare system.

Wrapping Up: The Value of the Reimbursement Roadmap

The reimbursement roadmap may seem complex, but it's a vital part of medical coding, ensuring that providers receive fair and timely payments for the care they provide. By understanding each step, from documentation to claim submission, coders can see the real-world impact of accuracy on both patient care and organizational stability.

As you continue coding, remember that every accurate code you submit not only reflects the care provided but also supports financial integrity, compliance, and the overall health of the healthcare organization. Each claim processed accurately is a step in the right direction for everyone involved, from the patient to the provider to the coder.

You're playing a critical role in the healthcare landscape, and your attention to detail makes a lasting difference. Keep up the great work—you're following the reimbursement roadmap to success!

Chapter 10

From Error to Expertise – Embracing Mistakes as Lessons

"Mistakes are the raw material of mastery. Each one carries a lesson, waiting to be uncovered and turned into expertise."

In medical coding, mistakes are inevitable. Even the most seasoned coders have stories of memorable errors that, while frustrating at the time, became valuable lessons. Coding is complex, detailed, and sometimes overwhelming, especially as you're learning. But each error holds a key to becoming a stronger, more accurate coder.

In this chapter, we'll talk about why mistakes are a normal part of mastering coding, how to embrace them as learning opportunities, and practical steps to turn them into moments of growth. Let's start with a story from my own experience—one that felt like a big setback at the time but ultimately shaped me into a better coder.

My First Big Error: A Lesson in Specificity

A few years back, I was working on a batch of outpatient claims for a group of surgical cases. One patient came in for what I thought was a straightforward procedure: a laparoscopic cholecystectomy, or gallbladder removal. The provider had documented the procedure thoroughly, and I coded it as I'd been trained—adding the basic CPT code for a standard laparoscopic cholecystectomy.

Fast forward a few weeks, and I found out that the claim was denied. I was confused; I had used the code I thought was correct. After checking in with my supervisor, we took a closer look at the documentation together. It turned out that the surgeon had documented additional work for a complex gallbladder removal due to severe adhesions, which required a higher-level coding. By coding it as a straightforward procedure, I had left out an important detail that impacted reimbursement.

This "mistake" became one of my best learning experiences. I learned to slow down, read through documentation thoroughly, and catch subtle notes that indicated a more specific or complex situation.

From then on, I made it a habit to look for any mention of added work or unusual circumstances. That one mistake taught me to prioritize specificity over speed, a lesson that has served me well in every coding project since.

Why Mistakes Are Essential to Mastery

Mistakes aren't just part of the learning process—they're fundamental to it. Coding is a nuanced, detail-oriented profession, and each error shines a light on areas where we can grow. Embracing mistakes helps you develop resilience, critical thinking, and a deeper understanding of coding guidelines. Here's why making—and learning from—mistakes is essential for growth:

1. **Mistakes Highlight Weak Spots**: Errors show us exactly where we need improvement, whether it's understanding a guideline, mastering a new code set, or paying closer attention to documentation.
2. **They Build Resilience**: Facing mistakes and learning to handle them without self-blame builds mental toughness, which is key in a field as detail-driven as coding.
3. **They Drive Continuous Improvement**: Each mistake gives us a chance to adjust our approach, improve accuracy, and develop better habits that contribute to long-term success.

Common Coding Mistakes and Lessons to Learn from Them

Let's look at a few common coding errors and the lessons they offer. Each mistake holds insights that can improve your coding skills and turn errors into stepping stones to expertise.

1. Missing Specificity in Diagnosis Codes

Selecting a general code when a more specific option exists is one of the most frequent errors coders make, especially in complex cases. This is often due to rushing or overlooking small details that hint at a more precise code.

- **Lesson**: Accuracy requires attention to detail. Take time to review documentation carefully, looking for keywords that indicate a specific condition, location, or severity. For instance, if documentation mentions "right lower quadrant abdominal pain," look for a code that captures both "right" and "lower quadrant" rather than a generic abdominal pain code.

2. Incorrect or Missing Modifiers

Modifiers are critical for providing extra details about a procedure, but they're easy to miss. Forgetting a necessary modifier can change the meaning of a code or lead to denials and underpayments, as modifiers often indicate complexity, laterality, or additional circumstances.

- **Lesson**: Develop a checklist for commonly used modifiers, especially in cases with multiple procedures. Taking a moment to verify that each procedure has the appropriate modifier can prevent issues and ensure accurate reimbursement. If you miss a modifier, use that as a reminder to check each one thoroughly next time.

3. Upcoding or Downcoding Due to Misinterpretation

Misunderstanding a guideline or overestimating the complexity of a procedure can lead to upcoding (choosing a higher-paying code than necessary) or downcoding (choosing a lower-paying code). These mistakes often come from a lack of experience with specific coding sets or misunderstanding of documentation.

- **Lesson**: When unsure, consult coding guidelines or reach out to a supervisor for guidance. If you discover you've upcoded or downcoded, take time to understand why the code was inaccurate and how to interpret similar cases in the future. Coding correctly isn't just about following rules—it's about understanding the intent behind the code.

4. Bundling Errors

Procedures that are bundled together per payer guidelines must be coded as a single package, but new coders sometimes code each element separately, leading to incorrect billing. This error often results from a lack of familiarity with bundling rules or payer-specific guidelines.

- **Lesson**: Review National Correct Coding Initiative (NCCI) edits and familiarize yourself with common bundling rules. If you encounter a denial for unbundled services, use that experience to dive into payer policies and adjust your approach accordingly. Bundling correctly ensures compliance and avoids denials.

5. Overlooking Documentation Clues

Sometimes the key to accurate coding is hidden in the details of documentation—details that can be easy to miss when you're working quickly or reviewing large volumes. For example, a phrase like "history of diabetes with complications" indicates the need for more complex coding than "diabetes."

- **Lesson**: Slow down and read documentation thoroughly, especially in complex cases. If you've missed a detail that led to an error, develop a habit of highlighting or noting critical phrases during your review process. Reading documentation like a detective makes coding both more accurate and more rewarding.

How to Embrace Mistakes and Turn Them into Growth

Making a mistake in coding can feel frustrating, but it's also an opportunity to build resilience and refine your approach. Here's a process for embracing mistakes and using them to fuel your development.

1. Acknowledge the Mistake Without Self-Blame

First, accept the error without being hard on yourself. Coding is complex, and no one gets everything right. Acknowledging the mistake without self-criticism helps you move forward constructively.

- **Practical Tip**: Remind yourself that every coder—no matter how experienced—makes mistakes. Shift your mindset from "I messed up" to "I'm learning."

2. Identify the Root Cause

Next, try to identify what led to the mistake. Was it a lack of understanding, a rushed decision, or a documentation issue? Understanding the root cause of an error helps you address it effectively and prevent similar mistakes.

- **Practical Tip**: Write down the reason for the mistake and keep a running list of common challenges. For example, if you miss modifiers frequently, make "modifier check" a specific step in your review process.

3. Consult Resources or Supervisors for Guidance

If the error stemmed from a knowledge gap, consult coding resources, such as the coding guidelines, National Correct Coding Initiative (NCCI) edits, or trusted coding references. If you're still unsure, ask a supervisor or experienced coder for advice.

- **Practical Tip**: Create a list of go-to resources, including coding manuals, payer guidelines, and reliable online references, so you can quickly address similar issues in the future.

4. Reflect and Adjust Your Approach

Each mistake presents an opportunity to adjust your process. Maybe that means adding a checklist step, slowing down when reading documentation, or making notes on specific coding guidelines. Adapting based on your errors makes you a stronger coder.

- **Practical Tip**: If you tend to make similar mistakes, develop a pre-submission checklist or create reminder notes for areas that need extra attention. These small changes build long-term accuracy.

5. Celebrate Small Improvements

Over time, you'll notice improvements in your coding skills thanks to the lessons learned from mistakes. Celebrate these small wins—they're proof that you're growing in your coding career and becoming more skilled every day.

- **Practical Tip**: Keep a "wins log" where you note improvements, successful coding audits, or new skills learned. Reflecting on your progress can boost confidence and motivate you to keep improving.

Building Resilience in Coding

Resilience is one of the most valuable traits in coding, and each mistake you overcome builds it further. Here are some ways to build resilience while embracing mistakes:

1. **Develop a Growth Mindset**: View each error as a learning experience rather than a setback. This mindset helps you stay open to feedback and motivates you to keep refining your skills.
2. **Create a Support Network**: Connect with fellow coders who understand the challenges of the field. Sharing mistakes, lessons, and tips with others helps normalize the learning process and makes coding feel less isolating.
3. **Practice Patience and Perseverance**: Coding accuracy takes time to develop. Be patient with yourself and remember that each day, you're gaining experience that will make future coding tasks easier and more accurate.
4. **Embrace Lifelong Learning**: Coding is a field where guidelines and practices change regularly. Embrace a mindset of continuous learning, knowing that mistakes are just part of staying up-to-date.

Wrapping Up: Turning Errors into Expertise

The journey from error to expertise is what makes coding both challenging and rewarding. Each mistake is an invitation to grow, to refine your skills, and to become more resilient. By embracing mistakes as part of the learning process, you're setting yourself up for a rewarding, long-lasting career in medical coding.

The next time you make a coding error, remember that it's just another step on your path to mastery.

With each mistake you learn from, you're becoming a more skilled and knowledgeable coder. Keep going—you're on the road to expertise, and every small improvement brings you closer.

Chapter 11

Charting Your Course – Building a Career Beyond the Codes

"Your career is more than a series of jobs—it's a story you're writing, chapter by chapter. Make each decision with intention, and let your journey inspire others."

Medical coding can be a fulfilling profession with ample room for growth, but there's more to this career than meets the eye. Coding skills are just the beginning. For those who are ready to move beyond the basics, the coding world offers opportunities for specialization, teaching, leadership, and consulting.

Whether you're just starting out or already experienced, this chapter is about exploring the pathways to a long and rewarding career, building a network, and continuing to grow professionally.

To make this journey personal, let me share a bit of my own story—a path that started with a desire to learn and eventually led to exponential growth.

My Journey from Non-Certified Beginner to Certified Professional

When I started as a coder, I didn't have any certification. I began as a non-certified fresher, and even when I shifted to a new company, I was still uncertified. I didn't realize just how much a certification could impact my career prospects. But as I gained experience, I saw more and more how certified coders were able to move into advanced roles, specialize in certain areas, and earn higher pay.

Determined to take the next step, I prepared for the

Certified Professional Coder (CPC) exam on my own, balancing work with study time and pushing through challenges. When I finally passed the CPC exam, I felt an incredible sense of accomplishment. This certification opened doors I hadn't thought possible before, and my career path transformed. With the CPC, I found opportunities for exponential growth that had felt out of reach before. These days, a CPC certification is often the minimum requirement just to enter the field, which shows how crucial it is for professional advancement.

Career Paths in Medical Coding: Charting Your Own Growth

Your journey in medical coding can go in many directions, and with each new skill and certification, doors open to new possibilities. Here are some common paths coders can consider for career growth.

1. Specialize in High-Demand Areas with Advanced Certifications

Specialized certifications allow coders to dive deeper into fields like inpatient coding, outpatient coding, or risk adjustment, which are in high demand. Specialization can enhance your earning potential, offer more job security, and enable you to work on complex cases.

- **Certifications to Consider**: AAPC and AHIMA offer certifications for specialties such as Certified Inpatient Coder (CIC), Certified Outpatient Coder (COC), and Certified Risk Adjustment Coder (CRC). These certifications set you apart and allow you to focus on areas of particular interest.
- **Example Path**: Coders who earn a CIC certification can work in inpatient coding, handling cases that require a detailed understanding of complex procedures and medical conditions.

2. Become a Coding Auditor or Compliance Specialist

If you enjoy accuracy and quality control, auditing and compliance could be a great fit. Coding auditors ensure that claims meet accuracy and regulatory standards, while compliance specialists focus on adherence to healthcare laws and guidelines.

- **Certifications to Consider**: Certifications like Certified Professional Medical Auditor (CPMA) from AAPC provide the knowledge needed to transition into auditing or compliance roles. This certification emphasizes compliance and auditing practices, preparing you to evaluate coding accuracy and maintain regulatory standards.
- **Example Path**: With CPMA certification, coders can join audit teams that review documentation, ensure compliance, and provide feedback to improve accuracy and quality.

3. Pursue a Teaching Role as an Approved Instructor

With the increasing demand for coding professionals, teaching offers a rewarding path where you can help prepare the next generation of coders. As an instructor, you can work in coding academies, training centers, or even teach remotely, sharing your knowledge and guiding others to success.

- **Certification to Consider**: Becoming an AAPC or AHIMA-approved instructor is a valuable credential if you're interested in teaching. These programs give you the certification and training needed to educate future coders and help them pass certification exams.
- **Example Path**: Approved instructors can teach in coding schools, healthcare organizations, or online platforms, giving back to the profession by preparing new coders and sharing their expertise.

4. Explore Healthcare Data Analytics and Informatics

For coders with a knack for data, healthcare analytics and informatics offer unique roles focused on interpreting data trends to support decision-making and patient care improvements. These fields often require analytical skills and a strong understanding of healthcare data.

- **Certifications to Consider**: Certifications like Certified Health Data Analyst (CHDA) help prepare coders for roles in data analysis and informatics, where they can transform coding data into actionable insights.
- **Example Path**: Coders with a CHDA certification may work in analytics roles, helping healthcare organizations identify trends, optimize patient care, and improve operational efficiency.

5. Step into Leadership and Management Roles

For those with strong organizational and interpersonal skills, management roles such as coding manager or team lead offer the chance to oversee teams, handle strategic planning, and ensure departmental goals are met. Coding managers take on responsibilities like quality control, team training, and setting productivity targets.

- **Certifications to Consider**: AAPC and AHIMA offer leadership-focused courses, as do healthcare administration programs. While formal management certifications aren't always required, courses in leadership or project management can be helpful.
- **Example Path**: Coders with experience and leadership skills can become coding managers, overseeing a team, implementing policies, and working directly with other departments to improve coding quality and compliance.

Steps for Professional Development and Growth

Professional growth is about more than just certifications—it's a continuous journey of learning, networking, and adapting. Here are practical steps to take as you chart your course.

1. Invest in Certifications that Support Your Goals

Certifications not only expand your knowledge but also show employers your commitment to the field. In today's market, certifications like CPC or COC are often minimum requirements for entry, while advanced or specialized certifications can propel your career forward.

- **Action Step**: Research certifications based on your interests. Begin with essential certifications like CPC if you're new, then pursue specialized or advanced certifications for targeted growth.

2. Build a Strong Professional Network

Networking connects you with other professionals, mentors, and potential employers who can support your career growth. Industry contacts can introduce you to new opportunities, keep you informed of trends, and offer valuable advice.

- **Action Step**: Join organizations like AAPC or AHIMA, attend industry events, and connect with professionals online. LinkedIn, coding forums, and AAPC community pages are great places to meet others in the field.

3. Stay Informed on Industry Changes

Coding guidelines and payer policies change frequently, and staying informed ensures that your skills and knowledge are current. Regularly reviewing updates keeps you adaptable and prepared for any coding changes that affect compliance and reimbursement.

- **Action Step**: Set aside time each month to review updates from sources like AAPC, AHIMA, and CMS. Being proactive helps you stay ahead and avoid coding errors due to outdated knowledge.

4. Develop Leadership and Communication Skills

Soft skills like leadership, communication, and problem-solving are essential if you're interested in roles like teaching, auditing, or management. These skills can be the difference-maker when advancing into supervisory or project management roles.

- **Action Step**: Take courses or workshops in leadership, communication, or project management. These skills prepare you for roles that require more than technical knowledge and are valuable in any professional setting.

5. Create a Portfolio of Your Work and Achievements

A professional portfolio is a powerful tool when pursuing promotions, new roles, or consulting opportunities. It showcases your certifications, accomplishments, project work, and any positive feedback you've received.

- **Action Step**: Start compiling certifications, letters of recommendation, project summaries, and performance reviews. Update it regularly to reflect your latest achievements.

Building a Professional Network to Support Your Goals

A strong network provides not only job leads but also support, mentorship, and insight into new trends. Here are ways to build connections that will help you advance in your career:

1. **Attend Conferences and Webinars**: Industry events provide both educational sessions and opportunities to meet other professionals. Whether online or in-person, these events offer valuable insights and connections.
2. **Join Professional Organizations**: AAPC, AHIMA, and local coding associations provide access to forums, training sessions, and networking events. Being active in these groups connects you with coders who share your goals.
3. **Engage in Online Coding Communities**: Platforms like LinkedIn, coding forums, and AAPC's community groups are great for sharing experiences, asking questions, and finding mentors. Participating in these communities helps you stay connected and informed.
4. **Conduct Informational Interviews**: Reaching out for a conversation with someone in a role you admire can provide insights and advice. These informal interviews help you learn from others' experiences and make valuable connections.

Setting Long-Term Goals and Staying Motivated

A career in coding offers the chance to grow in many directions, and setting clear goals will help you stay motivated and focused. Here's how to chart your course and make consistent progress.

1. **Define Your Vision**: Think about where you want to be in 5, 10, or 15 years. Do you envision yourself in auditing, teaching, leadership, or perhaps consulting?
2. **Break Goals into Manageable Steps**: Large goals can feel overwhelming, so break them down into smaller steps. For example, if you want to specialize in auditing, start by preparing for a CPMA certification.
3. **Celebrate Progress**: Each certification, promotion, or milestone is a step forward. Recognizing your achievements helps keep you motivated and reminds you of how far you've come.

4. **Seek Feedback and Adjust**: Regular feedback from mentors, supervisors, and peers is essential for growth. Use constructive input to refine your skills and stay on track.

Wrapping Up: Building a Career Beyond the Codes

Medical coding can be a lifelong career full of purpose, growth, and opportunities. By setting clear goals, building skills, and connecting with others, you can take coding from a job to a meaningful career path. Each certification, new role, and lesson learned adds to your journey, bringing you closer to your ideal career.

So, chart your course, embrace growth, and take steps toward the future you envision. Your journey in coding is just beginning, and every choice you make strengthens the foundation of your professional success.

Conclusion

The Art of Coding with Confidence

> "Confidence doesn't come from being perfect—it comes from knowing you can handle imperfections, learn from them, and keep moving forward."

As you reach the final chapter of this journey, take a moment to recognize how far you've come. Coding is more than just assigning numbers to diagnoses and procedures; it's a craft that requires precision, commitment, and a willingness to grow. You've tackled complex concepts, faced common "chief complaints," and learned how to navigate the challenges that coders encounter every day. With each chapter, we've delved into the realities of coding, from overcoming beginner mistakes and handling audits to embracing a career that offers endless learning and growth.

In this conclusion, let's reflect on the growth you can achieve by addressing these coding challenges head-on. The journey to mastery isn't about perfection; it's about embracing each experience as part of your learning path. You've already taken crucial steps in developing your skills and understanding that coding is a field where every detail matters—and every error can be a lesson that makes you stronger.

From Uncertainty to Expertise: The Growth You'll Achieve

Medical coding can feel overwhelming at times, with an ever-growing list of codes, guidelines, and regulations to remember. In the beginning, it's natural to feel unsure of yourself and to question whether you're truly cut out for this field. But as you've seen throughout these pages, each challenge—each "chief complaint"—is an opportunity to build confidence and competence.

Every coder, from the beginners to the veterans, has faced these hurdles and grown stronger because of them. By addressing common pitfalls like the "unspecified trap" or "modifier mayhem," you're learning to avoid errors that could lead to claim denials, lost revenue, or even audits. You've explored ways to embrace mistakes as learning opportunities and learned that ethical coding is not just a guideline but the foundation of your professional integrity.

Through practical strategies, this journey has prepared you to face the realities of coding head-on and to transform these challenges into strengths. By mastering these common coding complaints, you're on a path toward expertise, resilience, and a career filled with purpose.

Key Takeaways for a Confident Coding Journey

Let's revisit some of the most powerful lessons from this journey, so you can carry them forward as guiding principles.

1. Accuracy is Your Greatest Asset

- Accuracy isn't just about compliance; it's the bedrock of quality healthcare documentation and fair reimbursement. By double-checking codes, modifiers, and documentation, you prevent costly errors and help ensure that each claim reflects the care provided.
- **Remember**: Precision takes practice. Each time you review a chart or submit a claim, you're building habits that make accuracy second nature.

2. Mistakes are Stepping Stones to Mastery

- No one becomes an expert without making mistakes. Each error, from missing a modifier to selecting a non-specific code, is an opportunity to improve. Treat mistakes as stepping stones and view them as the valuable learning tools they are.
- **Remember**: Coding is a journey, not a race. Take time to analyze each mistake, adjust your approach, and trust that each lesson brings you closer to mastery.

3. Ethics are Essential to Professional Integrity

- Ethical dilemmas will arise, but the decision to code honestly and accurately is non-negotiable. Each time you code with integrity, you're protecting the healthcare system, the organization you work for, and, most importantly, the patients whose records you help maintain.

- **Remember**: Upholding ethical standards isn't just part of the job; it's a commitment to ensuring that coding remains a respected and trusted profession.

4. Growth is Ongoing

- Coding is a dynamic field where new guidelines, updates, and regulations are constant. Staying current requires continuous learning and a commitment to personal and professional growth. Certifications, workshops, and networking are tools that keep you informed and adaptable.
- **Remember**: Embrace lifelong learning. Whether it's earning a new certification or joining a study group, each step adds depth to your expertise.

5. Confidence Comes with Experience and Dedication

- True confidence in coding doesn't come overnight; it's built over time, with every chart reviewed, every guideline mastered, and every error corrected. Each coding choice you make adds to your confidence and builds a career founded on skill and resilience.
- **Remember**: Believe in your abilities and remember that every coder started where you are now. The small victories you achieve each day are building blocks for a future of expertise.

A Career of Purpose: Embrace the Path Forward

The art of coding is about more than the technicalities of codes and guidelines; it's about creating a career filled with purpose, integrity, and the desire to make a meaningful impact on healthcare.

Each code you assign is a building block in the larger picture of patient care, financial integrity, and healthcare documentation. The work you do matters—it supports fair reimbursement, ensures accurate patient records, and upholds compliance across the board.

Your journey in coding will bring new challenges, but with each one, you'll find that your skills, knowledge, and resilience are there to meet them. Your growth is a testament to your dedication, and as you move forward, remember that every coding decision you make contributes to the integrity of healthcare.

Final Words: Confidence, Mastery, and the Future

Mastery in coding isn't about knowing every answer—it's about having the confidence to approach each case thoughtfully, knowing where to find information, and trusting your ability to learn and adapt. The more you embrace each experience, the more you'll see coding as an art—one that blends skill, judgment, and a commitment to excellence.

You've embarked on a career that combines technical skill with ethical integrity, resilience, and continuous growth. This journey may not always be easy, but with every coding challenge you overcome, you're proving to yourself that you're capable of greatness. So keep learning, stay curious, and approach each new task with confidence. You're building a career that's not just about codes—it's about making a difference, one chart at a time.

Remember, coding mastery is a journey, not a destination. Every step forward counts, and every lesson you learn shapes the coder you're becoming.

Embrace the art of coding with confidence, and trust that your dedication and hard work are leading you toward a future filled with purpose, growth, and achievement. You've got this—your journey is just beginning, and the possibilities ahead are endless.

Glossary of Terms

A

- Abdominal Pain (R10.9): A generic diagnosis code used when the specific cause or location of abdominal pain is not documented.
- Acute: A term indicating a condition with a sudden onset, often severe in nature.
- Anatomical Terms: Words describing parts of the human body, such as cranial (skull), thoracic (chest), or femoral (thigh).
- Audit: A review process for evaluating the accuracy and compliance of coding practices.

C

- Chart Notes: Documentation by healthcare providers detailing a patient's symptoms, diagnoses, and treatment plans, critical for accurate coding.
- Chronic: Refers to a long-term or persistent condition, as opposed to acute.
- Coding Guidelines: Established rules and conventions for selecting accurate medical codes.
- Combination Code: A single code representing two diagnoses or a diagnosis with an associated secondary condition.

D

- Diagnosis Code: A code used to describe a patient's condition or reason for seeking medical care.

- Denial: A rejection of a claim by a payer due to errors or non-compliance in coding or documentation.
- Documentation: The written or electronic record of a patient's medical history, treatments, and outcomes.

E

- E/M (Evaluation and Management): A category of medical codes used for billing patient visits and related services.
- Excludes1: A coding guideline that indicates two conditions cannot be reported together.
- Excludes2: A guideline meaning the condition is not included in the code and may require separate reporting.

G

- Guideline Blindness: A term coined in the book to describe the oversight of coding conventions and standards.

L

- Laterality: A coding detail indicating the side of the body affected (left, right, or bilateral).

M

- Modifier 25: Indicates a significant, separately identifiable E/M service on the same day as another procedure.
- Modifier 59: Used to indicate a distinct procedural service when multiple services are provided.
- Modifiers: Two-character codes added to CPT codes to provide additional information about a service or procedure.

N

- National Correct Coding Initiative (NCCI): A set of rules preventing improper coding and ensuring compliance with standard coding practices.

P

- Principal Diagnosis: The main condition that prompted the patient's visit or treatment.
- Procedure Code: Codes used to describe surgeries, diagnostic tests, and other medical services.

S

- Sequencing: The order in which diagnosis or procedure codes are listed, affecting claim prioritization and reimbursement.
- Specificity: The level of detail captured in a medical code to reflect the precise nature of a diagnosis or procedure.

T

- TIA (Transient Ischemic Attack): A temporary period of symptoms similar to a stroke, caused by reduced blood flow to the brain.
- Tracking: Monitoring coding and documentation errors to improve accuracy and avoid repeated mistakes.

U

- Unspecified Code: A code used when documentation lacks sufficient detail for a more specific code.

V

- Verification: The process of checking documentation and codes to ensure accuracy and compliance.

W

- Workflow: The sequence of processes through which coding tasks are completed, including chart review, code selection, and claim submission.

www.ingramcontent.com/pod-product-compliance
Lightning Source LLC
LaVergne TN
LVHW091121150826
845673LV00002B/922

* 9 7 9 8 8 9 6 3 2 4 4 9 2 *